WOMEN AT RISK OF
*heart*_{*attack*}

March, 1997

To my friends the Arnolds,
With warmest wishes for your happy heart health and a salute to more happy times.
Mickey Hapner

WOMEN AT RISK OF

heart attack

A PERSONAL EXPERIENCE

A PERSONAL RESEARCH

by Mickey Wapner

Pangloss Press
MALIBU, CALIFORNIA

Copyright 1997
by Mickey Wapner
(All Rights Reserved)

Design by Joseph Simon
Composition by Greg Endries

From *Necessary Losses: The Loves Illusions, Dependencies, and Impossible Expectations That All of Us Have to Give Up In Order to Grow* by Judith Viorst. Published by Ballantine Books. Copyright © 1986 by Judith Viorst. This usage granted by permission of the author.

Library of Congress Cataloging-in-Publication Data

Wapner, Mickey, 1925–
    Women at risk of heart attack : a personal experience, a personal research / by Mickey Wapner.
       p. cm.
    Includes bibliographical references.
    ISBN 0-934710-35-X
    1. Wapner, Mickey, 1925 — Health. 2. Coronary heart disease — Patients — United States — Biography. 3. Women — Diseases. 4. Stress (Physiology) I. Title.
RC685.C6W37   1997
362. 1 ' 96123 ' 0092 — dc21
[B]   97-4454
                                                                           CIP

For Joe

ACKNOWLEDGMENTS

This is a very personal book, hence a very personal set of acknowledgments. This book is my life. My life is this book. Had many wonderful people not been there, I would not have lived to write it.

My first thanks go to my lifesavers, Dr. Carlos Blanche and Dr. John Bussell. In the surgeries, Carlos literally held my heart in his hands for an hour, bringing me back to life. John's brilliance and courage to experiment, brought life-saving anesthesia into my body. I felt from the very beginning that they were angels, doing God's work on earth. There have never been adequate words to thank them.

My family is and was my first line of defense. My beloved husband, Joe, children Fred, David and Sarah, Edna, Gabriel and Ariel, prayed and almost willed me back to life. My sister Berty, brothers- and sisters-in-law, Harry, Marilyn, Bernie and Nancy, sister-in-law and brother-in-law Irene and Russ, surrounded me and carried me forward through the mist of unconsciousness. And my friends, more numerous than I knew I had, kept the vigil and encouraged my recovery.

Leah Molle, who has been my life-long friend, admonished me to hang on and live, and stood by Joe. Dr. Bill Molle, my internist and friend of 45 years, took charge of my case and directed the huge medical team from my first report to him of trouble. And they spread their care and love to Joe. Dr. Harold Marcus performed angioplasty and stayed on my team till the end.

And then I started to write the book. First there were all the doctors who had a hand in the case, who gave freely of their recollections and medical information about my heart attack, cardiac arrest and recovery. My fullest thanks to my mentors: the late Ely J. (Jack) Kahn III of the New Yorker, and writer Eleanor Munro, his wife, who each told me how to get started—in exactly contradictory fashion; and to Rolando (Romeo) Hinojosa, a friend of our family from Mercedes, Texas, distinguished professor of English at the University of Texas, who encouraged me, gave me a crash course in writing, and read the first draft.

Special thanks to Dr. Grace Jameson, professor of Psychiatry at the University of Texas Medical School, who read the manuscript and said I had made a case for my life's stresses as a contributor to my heart disease.

And her daughter, Dr. Betsy Jameson, professor of history and women's studies at the University of New Mexico who read the manuscript with both a historian's and baby boomer's eye.

Rabbi Harold Schulweis counselled our family, gave me his pulpit so I could say thank you, and read my manuscript with enthusiasm and encouragement. He knows how late I came to God through my life's experience.

A special word of thanks to Judy Henteloff, who was my loving organizer and computer guide.

Thanks to my readers, Malka Schulweis, Frank Mankiewicz and Patricia O'Brien, Dr. Alvin and Marilyn Mars, Anne Berkovitz, Buff Given, and Mimi Perloff, who encouraged me to continue.

Thanks to Dr. Marianne Legato for her professional and personal endorsement of this book and for her introduction. And to Dr. Jack Matloff, whose genius built the cardiothoracic surgery unit at Cedars-Sinai Hospital and pioneered team medicine, and whose preface so carefully captures what motivated me to write.

And a special thanks to Joe Simon, publisher, of Pangloss Press, who loved the book, and told me not to change a word.

Contents

Foreword: Marianne J. Legato, M.D. 11
Preface: Jack Matloff, M.D. 13

Part One

1. A Journey of Discovery. 17
2. An Elephant Just Stepped On My Back 23
3. My Heart Attack 32
4. Complications 39
5. Looking for Answers 56
6. Witnessing Bypass Surgery 59
7. Stress: Long Term 71
8. Stresses of Early Life 79

Part Two

9. Matters and Myths of the Heart:
   The Gender Gap 87
10. Risk Factors and Warning Signs 98

Part Three

11. Marriage, Motherhood and Family 109
12. Travels with Joe 125
13. I am Now Older and Wiser 134
14. From Depression to Transformation 144
15. An Awakening 153

Part Four

16. What I Learned From My Heart Attack 161
17. What's In Store for the Next Generation 170
    Women's Statistical Table 173
18. Conclusion 176
    Afterword 181
    Selected Bibliography 185

foreword:
MARIANNE J. LEGATO, M.D., F.A.C.P.

Mickey Wapner's personal statement of the difficulties women face when they experience coronary artery disease is an invaluable contribution to women's health. Coronary artery disease kills a quarter of a million of American women annually; yet, breast cancer (which claims 48,000 lives a year) is what most patients fear.

Mrs. Wapner's description of what she suffered physically is not only gripping but medically accurate. Many questions physicians do not answer are addressed in this book, and will help patients who have had, or fear, coronary artery disease. Of particular value is Ms. Wapner's analysis of the role stress played in producing her heart attack. She observes, quite correctly, that most of the studies on stress and coronary artery disease have been done in men. The results cannot be extrapolated to women; women's interests, emphases and anxieties are for the most part very different than those of men.

This warm, personal and gripping account of how it feels to have and survive a heart attack will help the millions of women who have coronary artery disease, or who are at risk for it. Mrs. Wapner's passion to alert and educate American women about the major threat to their survival will benefit us all.

Marianne J. Legato, M.D., F.A.C.P. is an internationally known cardiovascular researcher, author, lecturer and specialist in women's health. She is an Associate Professor of Clinical Medicine at Columbia University College of Physicians & Surgeons and a practicing internist in New York City.

In 1992, Dr. Legato won the American Heart Association's Blakeslee Award for the best book written for the lay public on cardiovascular disease with her publication of the *The Female Heart: The Truth About Women and Heart Disease*, published by Simon and Schuster.

Dr. Legato is the editor of *The Female Patient*, and is on the editorial board of *Cardiovascular Risk Factors*. She writes continuously for both the scientific and lay communities, and for two years wrote a monthly column, "Your Health," for *Woman's Day* magazine. She is a consultant for several multinational corporations and provides expertise in the area of women's health.

preface:
JACK MATLOFF, M.D.

For those of you who chose to spend the time joining Mickey Wapner in her "survivor's story," you will be rewarded in a way that you could not have imagined. Because of her inherent curiosity and intellect, Mrs. Wapner has been able to relive a life-altering experience that addresses so many of the questions that are never even asked, let alone answered in life. Through her storytelling, she evolves and grows to maturity by sharing her insights and her inner strengths with you. She is obsessed with the need to "pay back" and, in sharing with you her experience, her teachings and advice are far beyond what anyone could have anticipated she would "pay back."

Along the way, one cannot help but come to understand how pervasive the factors are that underlie an experience with heart disease. Mrs. Wapner's story clearly establishes the fact that the experience of heart disease is not an individual one, but one that affects the entire family. Hers is the perfect description of the evolution, from lack of knowledge to enlightenment. While she did not have an "out of body experience" in the usually-accepted sense of the term, she clearly was able to come to an understanding of the traumatic events that surrounded her emergency cardiac surgery by reconstructing from personal interviews and the records all that happened. The excitement of the writer in this case is superseded only by the real life experience which is embodied in the expression, "an out-of-body experience."

Beyond the story of her personal journey, which she so poignantly shares with us, Mrs. Wapner also addresses the issue of women's health care in the 1990's. There is an increasing literature on the experience of heart disease in women, supporting her conviction that the care of women is often less than it ought to be. Whether it is because there is uncertainty about the nature of their symptoms; whether it is the teaching that they experience in early life about the duties of being a wife and a mother; or whether it is simply the expression of gender bias in our society, it becomes quite clear that we still have much to accomplish in how we care for women.

The current changing environment surrounding health care in general is also addressed by her in a very subtle way. Her story quite clearly expresses the fact that in today's health care environment for any patient is better off having a friend who is a doctor than of having a doctor who is a friend. As subtle as the differentiation may seem at first, it is apparent that the art of giving of oneself is still a critical part of caring for the medical needs of another. Without realizing it, her telling of her story is replete with examples of how important it is to the physician caring for a patient to care about the patient.

Mickey Wapner's story, beginning in the 1950's, is a remarkable tale of how much our capability in medicine has grown.

Finally, for those who have the sensitivity to understand what motivates us in our care of those we love, Mickey Wapner's story of her experience with heart disease and near death, teaches us that we can best say "thank you" by living life well and by continuing to be of service to others.

JACK MATLOFF, M.D.
Founding Chairman, Department of Cardiothoracic Surgery,
Cedars-Sinai Medical Center, Los Angeles

Part One

Mickey Wapner's experience is the perfect description of the evolution from the lack of knowledge to enightenment.
                                                JACK MATLOFF, M.D.

I. a journey of discovery

Like most women, I spent my adult years worrying about breast cancer, and then I was blind-sided by a heart attack that almost killed me. No one had ever told me, nor did I learn from media coverage, that heart disease is the number one killer of women today. When I turned fifty and entered menopause, I wasn't told that my risks for heart disease increased dramatically.

When I had my heart attack, my emergency room hospital chart—and all the others during my three weeks hospitalization—start with "sixty-five year old female" followed by descriptions of my current medical status. Nothing more.

Surely there was more to me than the "sixty-five-year-old female" described in the medical charts. Or the 40-year-olds and 50-year-olds and 60-year-olds and 70-year-olds who preceded me and have followed me into the hospital emergency rooms across the nation. Many of them not as lucky as I, to survive.

I was taking hormones. I was taking a calcium supplement, aware of the risk for osteoporosis. I have a yearly mammogram and have my breasts examined regularly, and then out of left field a heart attack surprised me. The number one cancer killer for women is lung cancer, and the cause is from smoking, just as smoking is a major cause for heart disease in women. Breast cancer, though much dreaded, has a relatively high recovery rate if detected early, and a much greater awareness factor among women than heart disease. Credit for this widespread awareness goes to women, the American Cancer Society, women doctors and young doctors. Now, what women have done to make breast cancer a national concern must also be done for women and heart disease. While everyone knows heart disease is the number one killer of American men, few of us realize that it is also the number one killer of women.

When I recovered and began to question why I had a heart attack, I was left without answers. The search for answers is the reason for this book. My purpose in writing it is to help other menopausal and post-menopausal women ask themselves these questions and get the answers before unsuspected heart disease knocks them out as it did me. And to help begin making women and heart disease a subject of national concern.

When I asked "Why me?" it wasn't because I felt sorry for myself. Quite the contrary, I was indignant.

How come I didn't know that all aging women are at risk for heart disease?

How come I didn't know that all post-menopausal women are at risk for heart disease?

How come I didn't know that I should have been monitored for heart disease at the outset and as soon as I was finished with menopause?

How come I didn't know about how stress works in heart disease?

How come I didn't know that my risks as an aging woman was as great as my husband's?

How come I wasn't as aggressive when it came to my healthcare as I was in caring for my family?

And how come I didn't know that I was a typical woman at risk even though I'd had what was considered good medical care? I had symptoms that, in a man, would have called for a stress test.

All of us women can only live our lives according to the hand we are dealt. That's how we play the game of life, that's the way I lived my life. That is true of genetics, of course. But I have learned that we can substantially change our lives—the hand we are dealt—by asking the right questions, of ourselves, our families, our doctors. And ask them we must if we are to survive.

Yes, I was a sixty-five-year-old woman when I had an acute myocardial infarction—heart attack—and I thought I had taken pretty good care of myself. I exercised and walked regularly. I was fairly careful with my diet. I had regular physical check-ups. But none of it was enough. And while I received the best medical care, not even the finest doctors in Los Angeles were vigilant about monitoring me for heart disease. I was a woman, right? Heart disease is a man's problem, right? Well, thank goodness I lived to set the record straight.

My exercise was without understanding. What should I have been aiming for? What was the purpose of it? How should I have programmed myself? And what was my objective? How should I have been monitored? I never asked any of my doctors, merely reported to them, and generally got a pat on the back for work well done.

As to my diet, it certainly had its lapses, and when I "cheated" and ate red meats, cheeses, eggs and desserts, I rationalized that it was reversible when I went back to being careful. Never suspecting that I was depositing plaque on my arteries. I didn't know that changing my diet wasn't a "sometime thing." I had to change the way I ate. Never to be on a diet. Just to learn to eat healthfully. We're talking about lifestyle changes. It has to be done.

Menopause wasn't much talked about as I entered it. I didn't know that the natural production of hormones prior to menopause was a protection against heart disease. Even when I was put on hormone replacement therapy, I wasn't told this was one of the reasons. I thought it was strictly to control menopause symptoms, night sweats, mood swings, hot flashes.

When I had my regular medical check-ups, the doctor said my blood pressure and cholesterol numbers were all right. That seemed good enough for me. I didn't question what those numbers were or if the same numbers that were all right for a man were also all right for a woman. I didn't know any better and I trusted the medical establishment. I never had a stress test. While this is a routine procedure for older men who receive quality medical care, it was *never even suggested.*

Let me give you a bit of background on who I was before my heart attack. After college I married Joe Wapner, law student, when I was twenty-one years old. I married him and lived his life. That's what was appropriate at that time. I put my career on hold, I saw him through law school and into his career. We had three children, two of them only fourteen-and-a-half months apart, one eight years later. We did the same things other couples were doing, getting a house in the suburbs, a mortgage, juggling relationships with in-laws, launching and promoting his career—trying to make it in the post-World-War-II era. Our friends, our neighbors, were like us. We all worked hard at what we now call the American Dream. Many of us succeeded—at least in making the dream come true for our families.

But I think we women were paying a price we didn't know about at the time. So I had this husband. He had his career, and I got his heart attack. I worried about him and his heart and his cholesterol and his stress all these years; so did his doctors. Then, I got the heart attack.

Of course I loved him—still do. Of course I loved the life we led—most of the time. Of course I loved the startling course our lives took when he became the People's Court Judge on TV—mostly. Many women would and did envy me.

Flying first-class back and forth across the country, sometimes two or three times a month.

Being picked up in limousines.
Sitting in on press and radio interviews.
Waiting with Joe and other celebrities before we went on camera.
Buying lovely clothes so I'd look just right for the cameras or the events.
Where's the stress?
All of this life was his life, not mine. And the hectic schedule was both of ours. I didn't make the plans, set the schedule, plan my life. I went along. I was dressed as a public commodity. I was playing a role, and that wasn't what I thought of as *my* life. And, I got the same exhaustion without the same satisfaction.

My problem, my mind set, my psychological needs were such that I still harbored a fiercely unfulfilled need to be someone on my own, by my own talents, by my own strength, by my own will. Not as someone's wife. I loved his success for him. He thrived on it. But not for me.

As the years of traveling accumulated, the excitement wore thin. As the feelings of being an appendage grew, my fatigue increased. I told Joe I wanted to cut back on the travel. It held no rewards for me, only strain. All of this was his life, and I had to make it on my own, to blunt my professional aspirations, to tamp down the frustration of finding my identity only through my husband and children.

How come I didn't know that this strain was stress, and it was taking its toll?

In spite of my preference for privacy I have written a personal story about my life hoping this might explain why I got a heart attack. I'm not any more certain today than I was in 1990 exactly why it happened, but my purpose is to ask you if you can find clues in your own life—or in my experience—to help you chart a new course. The exploration was helpful to me in my recovery. Maybe it will be to you in preventing a heart attack.

We women have cared for the men in our lives and the children in our lives, some of us with great good humor, creativity and grace, others with mixed feelings, others paying the high price of divorce, frustration, bitterness, and lack of fulfillment. But as we aged, we should have been told that heart disease is a medical problem that women have and can succumb to as often as men do. After we worry about *his* heart, and *his* career, and *his* stress, look what happens to *us:* we are subject to the same disease we always thought was exclusively his. That should not be and it doesn't have to be. It's time to pay attention to ourselves, to raise questions, to raise Cain with our doctors if need be. If it sounds like a battle cry, a clarion call, it is.

Listen, ladies, this book is about what happened to me, and it can happen to you. I got into trouble and almost died because certain procedures were not recommended or made available to me because I was a woman.

I am not a physician. My observations and recommendations are based on personal experience and substantiated by extensive research listed in the bibliography. I feel I have a perfect right to suggest to any reader and any physician who cares to listen that certain tests and guidelines be put in place for women. I have been asked what right I have to write a book that appears to give medical advice. I'm not giving medical advice. What I am doing here is giving you the benefit of my experiences. I have made no prescriptions, only recommendations of the things I do. I want to tell you how I got to this point of wellness today. Let me help you get there, too.

Let me begin the story in the hospital and, perhaps, save you a trip there.

A woman is twice as likely to die after her first heart attack.

2. an elephant just stepped on my back

I took off my wedding rings and handed them to Joe. "I know I'll make it. I have too much to live for." Each of us forced a smile to reassure the other. Joe stroked my face with a familiar, loving touch and bent down to give me a gentle kiss. At that moment we didn't know if we would ever see each other alive again.

The nurses had paused in their rapid journey down the hall just long enough for our brief farewell. They pushed my gurney through the doors of the surgical suite, into the recovery room, and gently rolled me into the first bed. Waiting for me were two men I had never seen before who would become the two most important men in my life: Carlos Blanche, the cardiothoracic surgeon, and John Bussell, the cardiac anesthesiologist. John took a brief history, "because we have to go into surgery fairly urgently," and gave me a thumbs up sign.

"Don't do that, it's bad luck," I said. "It was the last thing I saw Robert Kennedy do at the Ambassador Hotel before Sirhan Sirhan shot him."

John's brown hair was partially hidden under his green surgical cap. His light brown eyes didn't flicker, but he raised one of his heavy arched eyebrows, looked at me quizzically, and gave a slight nod.

Then Carlos explained briefly that he would perform the cardiac bypass surgery. His freshly scrubbed hands would hold my heart and my life in the next hours.

As the nurses pushed me into the cold, white, brightly lit operating room, I thought I heard classical music on a stereo. John introduced the IV and soon I drifted off.

This was Tuesday, February 27, 1990 about 4:15 p.m. I had been in the hospital fifty-eight hours.

Just four days earlier, I had celebrated my 65th birthday. At dawn I had walked along the spine of the Santa Monica Mountains, enjoying the glorious sunrise and the clear, cold air. It seemed a joke that I had just qualified for Medicare as I stepped up the pace on my familiar three-mile route. Later that morning, my closest friends were giving me an elegant luncheon. And that night I would celebrate with my family at a *Shabbat* dinner at home. I couldn't have felt happier or healthier.

The next night, Saturday, Joe and I returned from a wedding and sat down together for a cup of tea. Suddenly, I felt a wide band of pressure across my back. I thought it was my hiatal hernia acting up again, so I left the table, took the usual medicines (with little relief), went to bed and willed myself to sleep. Sunday morning about 5 o'clock, the pain came crashing back. It felt as if an elephant balancing on one leg had landed on my back. I didn't want to bother Joe. He's a sound sleeper, doesn't wake up quickly or with a clear head and besides, I thought, I could handle this myself. I slipped out of bed, tiptoed past the guest bedroom where my visiting cousins from Lithuania were sleeping, closed the door to my office, and dialed my close friend and doctor Bill Molle.

I described the symptoms. He, too, thought I was having a hiatal hernia attack, and suggested I repeat the medication and sit up. then, almost in passing, he asked, "Are you sweating?"

"No," I said.

I followed Bill's instructions, took the medicine, propped

myself up in my office lounge chair, and tried to relax. The elephant wouldn't budge. Within fifteen minutes I began to sweat profusely. I stumbled to the phone and called Bill again.

"I'm sweating and I'm scared to death, Bill."

"You'd better meet me at Cedars-Sinai," he said in a soft, firm voice. In our forty-three years as friends and as doctor and patient, I had never heard that tone in his voice.

I didn't know at that moment that what saved my life was having a long-term and personal relationship with my private physician. Many women—even those who can afford it—don't see their doctors regularly, and would not have felt comfortable making that call. Then there are the medically disenfranchised, who have no one to call.

I went to Joe's side of the bed, touched his shoulder and said, "Honey, you'd better wake up, we're going to Cedars-Sinai."

Joe does not wake up quickly, but this morning he sprang out of bed at the sound of my voice and pulled on some clothes. We got into the car at six o'clock, and all I said to him was, "don't stop for red lights."

I was having a hard time breathing, and when Joe asked what was wrong, I said I couldn't talk. Just before we pulled into the emergency parking area, the pain spread from my back and down the back of my arms to my chest.

I collapsed into a chair in emergency.

The nurse on duty asked, "What seems to be the problem?"

"I think I'm having a heart attack," I said. Suddenly human angels in green were surrounding me, attending me. There were so many I couldn't have counted them, even if I'd had my wits about me. They were professional, friendly, reassuring, each doing a separate thing, never seeming to run into each other. The one closest to me was a young Irish woman doctor; next to her, a very young, clean-shaven man with a diamond earring in his ear. I then saw a courtly gentleman with a large open face, light brown eyes and dark hair. Turning slightly, I also saw a rumpled, grumpy-looking doctor with a salt-and-pepper short beard wearing gold-rimmed bifocals. I must have surrendered to them (did I have any choice?), but I also felt they would take care of me, make me feel better. Oddly enough, I don't think I had any thoughts about survival at that moment, but I was scared.

At each step in the treatment, they explained what they were doing: they gave me oxygen through a nasal prong, inserted a catheter into my veins, and injected nitroglycerin to ease my chest pressure and morphine to relieve back and arm pain. Also heparin to thin my blood. And another dose of morphine.

"It's not getting any better," I said.

I was given three more doses of morphine, then more nitroglycerin. I felt another deep, sharp, pressure in my back; then a few minutes later the pain eased off.

While all this was going on, someone asked which of two programs of treatment I wanted them to follow—TPA, or something else.

"I don't know the difference, you decide," I told them.
Joe, who was there with Bill, agreed to the TPA protocol, the newest treatment to try to dissolve blood clots forming in the heart. This was then a national experimental program, administered in exactly the same sequence in each hospital participating in the research.

TPA was started, and at minute to minute intervals, over the course of the next hour-and-a-quarter, additional doses of medication were given. The pain fluctuated, but mostly remained unrelieved. I gathered it wasn't working.

I kept hearing one doctor saying, "We've got to get that plaque out of there. It's fallen into a dangerous place."

Plaque? something that formed on your teeth? Something that you were awarded and hung on the wall? I had never heard that the hardened cholesterol and gunk on your arteries was called plaque.

I had now been in the emergency room three hours. Dr. Sandra Fallon, the young Irish doctor, explained the coronary angiogram procedure to me, and for good measure, she added angioplasty and "possible" cardiac bypass surgery. I felt morphine groggy, but apparently expressed enough understanding to consent to the next phase of treatment.

I was wheeled into the catheterization lab. A gray-haired nurse told me she was going to shave my pubic hair, but not to worry, it would grow back.

"At my age?"

She smiled and nodded at me.

Although slightly dazed, I was alert enough to follow what was going on around me. And Bill and Joe were at my side to interpret. By this time, I don't know how many catheters I had in me or how many fluids were dripping through the lines, but now another little cut was made, high up in my right groin, another catheter was inserted, and a thin wire tube threaded up through the artery into the right side of my heart.

"We're taking a look in that area," said Harold Marcus, the rumpled, grumpy doctor who had been called in for the first phase of treatment and stayed by my side. He told me he expected the disease to be in the left coronary artery, but that he wanted to make sure the right one was unobstructed.

Everything on my right side seemed normal, but, as they suspected, the main artery on the front of my heart (the left anterior descending) was from 90% to 100% closed. The clot and some broken pieces of plaque had fallen against the diagonal that forms a v-shaped intersection with this main artery.

This position was what prompted Dr. Marcus to say over and over, "We've got to get that plaque out of there." This quick and extraordinary diagnostic procedure showed the doctors the location and severity of the problem. I had suffered an acute myocardial infarction—a severe heart attack—and the TPA had not dissolved the clot.

The next step was balloon angioplasty, a precise method of attempting to open a channel through closed arteries, to let blood flow through by squashing the collected plaque, like a roto-rooter going through clogged plumbing lines. To begin with, they made a cut in my groin and threaded a thin wire up through an artery into my heart. Now one wire tube was threaded inside another, and then another inside of this hollow, straw-like wire, and another wire thread with a very strong balloon attached to the end. A series of balloons were then inserted and inflated, each slightly larger than the last until the artery was forced open. This first procedure opened the artery about forty percent. As soon as the opening was sufficiently enlarged, I felt instant relief from the pain. It was exhilarating to be able suddenly to breathe.

"She was the least likely of my patients to have a heart attack," I heard Bill telling the team. "She ate sensibly, didn't smoke, wasn't overweight, walked three miles a day."

"Under any stress?" someone asked.

At that point I was sent to the Cardiac Intensive Care Unit on the fifth floor. The nurse kept reminding me to keep my leg straight at all times. "I don't want you to disturb the sheath and sand-bag weight we put on your leg. It's for pressure against the catheter in your femoral artery where we opened you up for angioplasty," she said.

I felt uncomfortably hot and aware of a dull pain in my lower back. Then came nausea and vomiting. But before I went to sleep that first night, I felt fairly comfortable.

I spent a restless night—bouts of nausea, vomiting, headaches, a dropping blood pressure, and some disturbance in the rhythm of my heart. At 5:30 Monday morning I asked the nurse, "Am I going to make it?"

"Don't worry, dear, we're taking care of you," she said.

I had uncontrollable chills and a spastic colon pain. I was given additional medications by supportive nurses. Quiet professional talk, soft squeezes of the hand, pats on the shoulder, gentle massages for my aching body, and prompt attention to each change and emergency were reassuring.

The day passed uneventfully; there were recurring moments of nausea and several episodes of that band-like pain in my back, but all of this was relieved with medication. While my son Fred was visiting me in Intensive Care, Dr. Marcus came into my room and ripped a few pages off the daily calendar, glanced at the electric clock that had stopped, muttered something unintelligible, left the room abruptly, and returned with a battery for the clock.

"You can't tell night from day in this place," he said, "so we have a calendar and clock to keep the patient oriented."

He then asked a nurse to get him a certain portable machine for further diagnosis; he waited a few moments, mumbled to himself, and disappeared again. A few minutes later he pushed the machine into my room fifteen steps ahead of the exasperated nurse. My son Fred and I shook our heads with disbelief.

"If that's the way you act at home, I feel sorry for your wife," I told Dr. Marcus.

I was still scared, trying to take in the nurse's explanations about the medications that were dripping into my veins along with their warnings to lie still and not to lift my head.

Late Monday night, Dr. Marcus told me he would decide the next day what to do. I wondered what that might be, but as I tried to sleep, worries about my family crept in. Their anguished faces flashed before my eyes. Was Joe as confident as he acted? How was Fred going to pull himself together? I hated adding this burden to David and Edna, my son and daughter-in-law, as they planned their move to Israel. Was my daughter Sarah, with her congenital heart condition, identifying with me? I hoped they could keep this news from my failing eight-seven-year-old mother-in-law and my near-senile mother.

The next day, Tuesday, at two o'clock in the afternoon, Dr. Marcus came in to remove the artery and venous lines.

"I plan to remove the clamp and start the heparin drip again in about an hour-and-a-half," he said.

Before he could do that, however, pain exploded in my back, exactly in the same place and with the same severity. The elephant had jumped again. Again, I was given more nitroglycerin in an attempt to relieve the pain. Again, a conference between Joe and Dr. Molle. I knew they were meeting and I couldn't imagine what was taking so long. I was getting more and more anxious and glad to see Joe come in.

"Honey, we've had two conferences; one with Dr. Marcus and one with Dr. Blanche," Joe said. "At first, Dr. Marcus wanted to do another angioplasty, but we ruled that out since the first one didn't work. I asked for a consultation with Jack Matloff who is the head of cardiac surgery and just came back from sabbatical; but Dr. Marcus said, 'Jack Matloff has built a great team here. Go with the guys on duty.'"

I lay still and quiet, trying to take it all in through my pain, stupor from the medications, fatigue from the heart attack and failed angioplasty and stark fear.

Joe said, "Dr. Blanche has studied your charts and he doesn't like what he's seeing on the monitor—another heart attack on the way. He told me there wasn't much time to spare and recommends you go in for surgery as soon as possible. You know they'll need your consent before they proceed," he said as he stroked my hand.

"Okay, Okay, let's get on with it," I said.

At 6:40 Tuesday evening the operating room nurse came to take me into surgery. Just before they pushed me into the operating room, Leah, Bill Molle's wife, shook her finger in my face and said, "You've got to make it for me." I was wide awake, full of pain, bewilderment and anxiety. None too soon, Dr. John Bussell connected the lines to catheters already in place, introduced new ones, and sent the anesthesia into my body. The most important hours of my life were underway.

And how come I didn't know I was the typical woman at risk?

3. my heart attack

What had triggered my totally unexpected, out-of-the-blue heart attack?

Looking back at my medical history, and Joe's, we didn't get treated unequally or badly considering our squeaky clean medical pictures. There were no clues. Up to the moment it happened, I felt wonderful, grateful beyond measure for my good fortune. It was also true that I had just completed the most strenuous year of my life, and that in spite of a glorious trip to Australia and New Zealand, I was bone tired. Within three days of our return from New Zealand, I had unpacked, gone to the cleaners, the beauty parlor, repacked, and taken off again for Phoenix, Arizona to attend a tennis tournament. This whirlwind was typical for Joe and me.

From the time Joe was chosen to be the Judge on the nationally syndicated television program, "the People's Court," the public part of our lives had changed dramatically. Being invited to participate in celebrity tennis tournaments was one of the perks Joe enjoyed tremendously. The only one I liked was the Senators Cup, because the players reminded me of my own political life. For sixteen years, John Gardiner had invited Democratic and Republican U.S. Senators along with national business leaders and a few celebrities to compete in a fundraising tennis tournament. So, going there three days after a major trip hadn't seemed like a strain.

Four days later, we flew from Phoenix to New Orleans for the annual meeting of the National Association of Television Production Executives (NATPE), the gigantic national gathering of television program purchasers who come to meet with the talent, producers and distributors to buy shows for the next season.

The cavernous convention center throbs with music. Brilliant light shows, glitz and glitter, flowers, plants and bunting decorate booths of the major and many minor TV distribution companies. Guests can eat their way from appetizers to ice cream as they crowd through the halls. One might rub shoulders with Dr. Ruth Westheimer, Michael Douglas, someone dressed like Bugs Bunny or Batman, a wrestler, Candace Bergen, Jesse Jackson, and less familiar TV network and production executives. Joe as part of the talent, was invited to spend time in the booth to meet television exhibitors from around the country, have his picture taken with them, sign autographs.

The first year we had gone to NATPE, the meeting was held in Las Vegas. At the distributor's private party, Joe and I were dancing when a woman tapped me on the shoulder and asked, "Mind if I cut in?" I was left open-mouthed, stranded in the center of the floor as she danced off with my husband. Shortly afterward, a waitress came up to Joe to say that she and her husband watched him everyday and bet on each of his decisions. For me, it was "Welcome to Las Vegas, and welcome to your new life" rolled into one. I wasn't sure I was going to like it.

At first I stood by Joe's side, and he introduced me to each person who came by. People would turn aside, sometimes mumbling a word of acknowledgment, and look at the place where I was standing as if it were vacant. Women frequently shouldered their way between Joe and me. Gradually I retired to the rear of the booth, and then decided not to come to the convention floor; instead I could explore the city, the region.

It had taken a long time, but by 1990 I felt little resentment, and it was a way to protect myself.

We came home to L.A. to our usual flurry of activity, and to make final arrangements for my Lithuanian cousins, who were to arrive on February 6th.

We found them in 1988 when we went to the Soviet Union to visit refuseniks, Jews who had been refused permission to emigrate from the USSR. My first contact with my cousin Elzbieta Z. Staskeviciene was by cable, introducing myself, telling her we would be in Vilnius, and would like to see her. Plain, flat cable language. Their response was the same, they would like to see us. In those few words a floodgate of emotion was unleashed on two continents.

After a frustrating night of canceled flights and waiting in the Leningrad airport lounge for five hours with no food, drink or information, we arrived in Vilnius bleary-eyed, exhausted and still feeling the stress of looking over our shoulders for the KGB. Nothing could have prepared me for the sight we saw in our hotel lobby when we walked into an assembled group of six first cousins, some of them with their children and grandchildren. For a moment we stood timidly apart. As I looked from face to face, I saw my mother, my Aunt Toby, my Aunt Annie, my Uncle Louie—the familiar features of my family on those faces. Then they surrounded Joe and me in embrace, and we sobbed for the years that had passed, and for the family history we had not shared.

We spent only one day-and-a-half together. In those hours, we drove across Lithuania and across time to cousins' homes in Kaunas and sixty miles to Uzvent, my mother's birthplace. We walked into mother's weathered wooden home; we walked the unpaved village streets she had walked as a child; we climbed a hill to the cemetery where my great-grandparents were buried. My roots were deeper there than I had known.

We walked past the houses where my grandparents, my

aunt and uncle and their five children had been tortured, and, into the forest where they were shot and buried in a common grave by Lithuanian Fascists. There I placed a rose and I recited the *Kaddish* (Jewish memorial prayer) over what had to pass as their grave.

Within a few hours of meeting them Joe asked who would like to come and visit the United States. Three hands shot up, Antanas, Elzbieta, and her son Raimondas. This remnant of my Lithuanian family were the cousins who were sleeping in my home the night of my heart attack.

A few months after our return home, I invited them to visit us. What I didn't know until they arrived (through a translator), was that they had requested a visa for two months, just in case they wanted to travel around the country, and that they were each able to bring only $300. In their naiveté, they expected they might be able to work here and earn some money. Joe, feeling manipulated and not in charge, began to fidget in his soul, which always shows in his body, but he left the arrangements to me. I shifted into high gear. I found a number of translators. I put together a dynamite, almost exhausting schedule for their visit.

So what began as Joe's throw away line in Elzbieta's living room in Kaunas in September, 1988, and an invitation from us to come for three weeks in October, 1989, stretched out to a sixty-three day visit. I remembered what James Beard said about guests, like fish, "After three days they smell." What about sixty? I was about to become a prisoner of the past I so very much had wanted to reclaim.

A family delegation went to the airport to greet them on February 6, 1990.

My appointment book was written in black or blue ink (for me), with the cousins' schedule in purple. Calendared in purple ink for the first eighteen days I had scheduled twenty activities, from supermarket visits, to Disneyland. It was like having children all over again. I took care of them as I had taken care of my children. They were unsophisticated, charming, likaeble, and totally dependent on me. I felt I had an obligation not only to show them but to teach them. The way I went about it, the sense of pressure on me mounted.

I was on duty every day. Everywhere I drove them I told the history and sociology of the area. In addition to the regular tourist attractions of Southern California, I felt it was important for them to see the ethnic diversity and spectrum of economic circumstances of our population: Koreatown, Chinatown, South Central Los Angeles, Hispanic communities, both old and new, early California bungalows, mansions in Bel Air.

To try to dilute the impact of the comparative privilege we enjoyed, I told them our family stories: how mother had sacrificed and worked as a housemaid when she first came here; how Aunt Toby had lived in back of her store with Uncle Jack when they were first married. As we passed the homeless sprawled in doorways and along city sidewalks, I explained how this tragic phenomenon had so recently spread like cancer across our whole country. Of all the things they saw and did, this made the greatest impression on them.

At the same time, we also tried to keep up with our own other appointments and obligations. Every day Joe would feel crowded, imposed upon, and though he often kept to his own schedule while I saw to the cousins' activities, their visit was clearly beginning to wear on him as well as on me. Things came to a head on the sixteenth day of their visit, as Joe and I drove across town to a wedding about an hour's drive from home, a perfect amount of time for conversation. Two people held captive in the car; there is no escape, except the radio. I chose to bring up the cousins' visit, to go over the schedule I had arranged.

It all started innocently enough, my aim was merely to plan ahead. I asked Joe how we might go about the next few days. His reply was swift, loud, emphatic: he erupted. Joe was laser hot and furious, told me he felt trapped, taken advantage of, and did not want to have any part of their remaining visit. He resented having to pay all their expenses, he was furious that they were taking advantage of us, and he was not going to do any more for them. He had done all he was going to do. He was not going to have his life ruled by them for the next forty days, and if I wanted to devote myself to it, knock myself out, it was okay with him, but he was washing his hands of the whole thing.

I asked, I begged for help. He said no.

"Can't you accept that they're here, and do the best we can?" I screamed.

He ground his teeth, clenched his fists on the steering wheel. "You can do what you want to with them, I'm finished. I'm washing my hands of the whole thing."

I could hardly believe my ears. "It's unfair of you; after all, it was your idea, you're the one who invited them here."

"I've done as much as I'm going to do. We've spent all this money and that's enough. I'm finished." he said.

I guess we screamed at each other for twenty miles. And then he clammed up. There was no more conversation.

And we were at the wedding. At the moment he opened his door to get out, I knew I would have to compose myself, put on my public face, smile and be a proper wedding guest. I was accustomed to that; hadn't I been living most of my life that way?

But something happened to me that had never happened before. My body contracted inside of me. I went rigid. I felt pressure inside my chest cavity and contractions gripping my stomach. I felt as if my blood pressure was shooting up, my stress level at overload, and I wanted to take flight. But all I could do was stay in place. Then I felt as if glass was breaking, crashing, cascading down into some chasm, but I didn't have time to pick up the pieces or try to put them together.

What I most wanted, or thought I needed, was a good stiff drink. There was no bar in sight. I smiled and moved toward the wedding patio. I did what I had done so many days in my life, put the lid on my feelings. Smash them down. Crush the inclination to run away, to scream out in pain. No. Put on a good face. Be a good girl. The years of practice had served me well. The pain subsided, the glass stopped breaking. Friends came to visit, newly introduced persons engaged me in conversation.

Three or four hours later, we were on our way home. I don't remember if we spoke, probably not, there was nothing to say. Joe had made a pronouncement. I knew I had the capacity and pride and determination to pull off managing the cousins' vacation without him. My fury and resentment at being told once again to operate on his agenda only fueled my determination to overcome the handicap. I would do what I had always done, throw myself into the project with good humor, steely resolve and pride. Underneath, the boiling cauldron would simmer, but the lid would be on. I would do it, I would triumph. I would put on a pleasant face, even to Joe, and keep on living.

A few hours later, more relaxed and easier, we sat down for a cup of tea, and the elephant stepped on my back, the band of pressure and pain crossed my back, sending me to bed.

"If a woman gets a heart attack, she is twice as likely to die within the first weeks as a man, and twice as likely to have a second attack within a year." — Marianne Legato, M.D.

4. complications

It was the evening of February 27, two days after my heart attack. At this point I had been in surgery three hours, undergoing double bypass surgery. The last two days had been the worst of my life—impossible to describe.

By 1:00 p.m. the surgery was complete. At 10:30 p.m. Dr. Carlos Blanche came out all smiles and said, "The surgery went very well, no complications. There's no reason for concern, everything is going to be fine."

"Can I see her?" Joe asked.

"Yes, but she's completely out, very cold and still blue, and she doesn't look very good," Carlos said. "Go home and get some sleep. I'll only call you if there's some emergency."

The family, reassured, left the hospital.

At 11:00 p.m. I was admitted to the Cardiac Surgery Intensive Care Unit, (CSICV). Carlos signed the post-operative orders and went home. John dropped into bed like a fireman, with his clothes close to the bed.

At 11:35 a Code Blue was called. My heart was fibrillating, I had suffered a cardiac arrest. No heart beat. No brain waves.

The Code Blue team, on call at all times, responds to the area where the call originates. The team carries a life pack of appropriate emergency equipment.

In the meantime, a physician in the CSICU had sent an emergency page, summoning each member of the surgical team. A doctor from the hospital paged Carlos, telling him I had gone into cardiac arrest.

By the time the team returned, the cardiac surgery Fellow (a physician in final hands-on specialized training) on duty at my bedside had opened my chest, removed the sutures, cut through the fresh stitches on two levels of skin, and cut through the heavy wires that Carlos had twisted into place just minutes earlier. There was a moment of tension with the nurse on duty who said the Fellow had no business doing that, it was Carlos' responsibility and only his. When he rejected her admonition, she walked off the case. Another nurse quickly took over.

It took Carlos fifteen minutes to be at my bedside. He was faced with a situation where the Fellow had opened the chest in the CSICU with no surgical technique, no sterility, just a few towels around the incision. He put on gown and gloves and began to massage my heart, which was basically gone—it was blue and was not contracting.

Carlos gave me all the medications called for in such a situation. Medications to make my heart beat. Medications to stop the irregular rate. He defibrillated me many, many times with small paddles that carried strong electric currents directly to my heart and with other shocks from outside the chest. At the same time, he was busy with his right hand massaging my heart, strong squeezes, fifty, sixty, seventy times a minute, simulating the regular heart beat, trying to provide some circulation to the brain. ("The heart can take some insult," he told me later, "but not the brain. The brain needs blood pressures. You may salvage the heart but the brain is gone if there is no blood. Looking at the screen there was not much blood pressure and no blood volume there; the only thing that was good, the temperature was pretty low.")

The team worked on me for an hour or more with no apparent results. The heart would not come back. Later, Carlos told me: "We gave medications directly into the heart, the veins, everywhere. We gave you oxygen, 100% oxygen, and we shocked you many times, but the heart just would not come back. An hour was more than a reasonable time; usually we work for about twenty or thirty minutes and if we see some signs of the heart coming back, we keep going. If not we just give up.

"In a situation like this you don't take the decision upon yourself," he said. "You ask around—nurses, technicians. Luckily, at that moment John Bussell came in. I told John I thought we should give up because it had been an hour and your heart wasn't showing any signs of coming back."

In response to Carlos' request for the team's ideas, John asked if he could try some things.

"Sure," Carlos said.

John told me later: "I used a very large dose of nitroglycerin intravenously. Your blood pressure was already very low, virtually nonexistent. Nitroglycerin at that dose would lower a normal blood pressure to that range, so if your blood pressure was sixty, seventy, eighty, I would never have advocated trying something like that. But since your pressure had been down there for so long, and since it seemed like there was no downside risk to it, I gave a large dose of nitroglycerin in the neck catheter, so it went right into the heart. An effect of the nitroglycerin is to dilate the heart or coronary arteries. My thought was that if for some reason, there wasn't enough blood supply to the heart and that was why it wasn't pumping—perhaps from a spasm of a coronary artery occurring spontaneously even though you've had bypass grafts—then nitroglycerin might help."

John now asked the team how much calcium I had received. The dose had been somewhat small, so he gave me additional calcium. Carlos massaged the drugs around my heart to get them to work. John decreased the amount of some of the drugs

I was receiving to raise my blood pressure because they weren't achieving the desired effect.

At that moment, the lab report on my arterial blood gas came back. The oxygen level was respectable, because of Carlos' massaging and ventilation, and the carbon dioxide level, though not normal, was not too bad. What was unusual was that there was very little circulation in removing the waste products of metabolism from my blood.

John said to the team: "If you gave me this blood gas and this patient, I would have said, they're both horrible, but they don't go together; this blood gas is better than this patient looks, and since I can't reconcile it, let's work a little harder, do a little more and see if we can get either one to be better. They should match."

"This isn't conventional cardiopulmonary resuscitation, Dr. Bussell," one of the cardiology Fellows said to John.

"We're way beyond conventional anesthesiology here, son," John said.

In the next five minutes, my blood pressure came back, my heart rhythm came back. The team waited in the intensive care for about fifteen minutes to see if I would remain stable. Then I was taken back to the operating room. Again, I was put on the heart-lung machine, the blood drained from my body and recirculated through the machine, allowing Carlos the opportunity to evaluate the condition of the bypass grafts. The bypasses were open and functioning.

Carlos assessed the situation as the team re-assembled in the operating room, and faced two problems. As he told me later, "We didn't know if your brain was working because the blood pressure was very low, and I wasn't sure we could get the blood circulating to the brain at all. The second problem was infection, because basically there were no precautions for infection, a few towels here and there, and almost bare hands inside the chest, and everybody in the room looking inside. The CSICU is not a sterile place. In the operating room, we saw what we had: the heart was coming back, but not strong enough."

Carlos opened my left groin and inserted an intra-aortic pump to assist my heart. It was beating reasonably well, and the blood tests and chemistries were normal at that point. He could not figure out what had happened, so he flushed the open cavity with a slush of ice and water, siphoned out the water and diluted blood, put in antibiotics and removed the clamps that spread my rib cage apart. Then he threaded the heavy wires through my ribs and pulled the rib cage together, threaded the wires across the separated portions of my sternum, twisted the wires together, sewed my dermis and then my epidermis together with a tiny curved needle. The operation took three hours.

"We closed," Carlos told me later, "But I was honestly not optimistic about it. I said to myself, 'Well we saved the heart, but that's pretty easy to do sometimes. The heart is working, but what good is it if the brain is not working?' And then I thought it was just a matter of time before the infection would show up."

Dr. Peter Chang Sing, the cardiovascular surgeon who had opened my chest in CSICU, called Joe at 1:30 a.m. to tell him that I'd had cardiac arrest, that they had to open me up. Joe should return to the hospital immediately, Carlos wanted to speak to him. In the meantime, Carlos called Bill Molle. Again, Joe drove through the city in the dark of the night. Again, he raced through red lights.

"All I could do was to hold on to the wheel and look straight ahead and say, 'You gotta save her. You gotta save her, you gotta save her.' Who I was talking to, I don't know, but I said 'You gotta save her,'" Joe told me later.

Joe got to the hospital, raced up to the sixth floor. It was empty. Almost crazy with dread, he tried to phone the doctor who had called. Dr. Sing finally came to talk to Joe to tell him what had happened and said Carlos would be out as soon as he could. About five minutes later, Bill and Leah came to sit with Joe.

At 3:30 a.m. Carlos came out, ashen faced, his dark eyes troubled. This time was entirely different than it had been at 10:30 p.m. the night before. He laid out the entire scenario of what he thought was happening: that I had experienced ventricular tachycardia (irregular heart rhythm), which soon went into malignant arrhythmias (life threatening irregular heart beat) and then ventricular fibrillation—in other words, where my heart stopped, had no regular contraction, was not beating in any orderly fashion, just quivered like a bowl of jello. He explained the attempts at emergency life-saving procedures, and the just-concluded second surgery. He was joined by the technician who had inserted the intra-aortic balloon pump to control the heartbeat. Carlos did not give Joe and Bill and Leah much hope.

"It was very grim—very grim," Carlos said. "She might not pull through." He told Joe to go home, he would be in touch.

Bill signed the hospital records, "Prognosis guarded."

I was wheeled back to CSICU in stable condition, cold and comatose. Carlos sat by my bed for several hours with very little hope for his patient.

Leah wanted Joe to go home with them, but he said he'd rather be at our home. It was now four in the morning. Sleep would not come to him in those pre-dawn hours, and by six-thirty, he got out of bed and called our children, Fred and David and Sarah, to tell them what had happened in the early morning hours, crying, "It doesn't look good, it doesn't look good."

It did not take them many minutes to come back home to their father's side. Again, trips across town in the early dawn. Fred arrived, fell into Joe's arms, burst into tears and told his father he should have called him the minute he knew, so he could have come to be with him. Sarah called her work and said she would not be in. David flew out of the house leaving Edna to explain to their two small boys that Grandma Mickey had taken a bad turn. As each of them arrived, Joe fell into their arms sobbing, the first time any of them had seen him cry since the heart attack.

"I'm scared. I'm scared," he said. "The doctors don't know if she's going to make it, and if she does, there's a good chance she'll have some brain damage. It just can't happen. It just can't happen to this woman."

Family and friends gathered. Our rabbi came to offer comfort.

Meanwhile, at the hospital, hour after hour, all morning and into the afternoon, I lay still, unmoving, unaware of the activity swirling around my bedside. Many times they squeezed, pinched me, stuck me with needles. No response.

Within twenty-four hours, after two operations, Carlos told me later, most patients would be waking up a little, but I had almost no brain activity. I was not responding to the painful pinches, squeezes, needle pricks. I was totally dependent on the respirator and the intra-aortic pump. There was no movement, no respiration. After they delivered me to CSICU at 3:30 a.m., I warmed up gradually, but nothing changed. At 7:30 a.m., the nurse noted that I remained unresponsive, without movement, or reflexes, the pupils of my eyes remained dilated, and I was only sluggishly reactive to light. Bill Molle came to the same conclusions on his early morning visit.

At 11:00 a.m. Dr. Marcus wrote in his report, "Catastrophic event of this early morning reversed. Patient currently hemodynamically stable in sinus rhythm, but, unfortunately remains deeply comatose and unresponsive. It is uncertain how much is due to neurological damage and how much to residual anesthetic and neuromuscular blocking drugs. I suggest early involvement of neurological consultants."

At 11:30 a.m. Carlos noted, "She is comatose and unresponsive, even to painful stimuli. Agree to neurological consult, but prognosis at this point looks grim. Husband informed."

At 1:30 p.m. I opened my eyes. I had been in a coma for fourteen hours.

The nurses and doctors in CSICU noticed that I seemed responsive. "Patient may have understood the command to close her eyes." The nurse said I opened my eyes and blinked on command. Carlos was in surgery. John walked in and said, "She's moving." He went to CSICU and administered additional drugs which would reverse, or counteract, any residual anesthesia effects so that a clearer picture of my neurological status could be ascertained.

At 2 o'clock Dr. Richard Gray, associate cardiologist of the cardiac surgery unit, called Joe and said, "I think your wife is coming out of the coma."

"Can I see her?"

"No, not yet. Let's wait a little while and see what else happens."

But Joe released his pent-up emotions, and let out a scream, "She's waking up!"

At 4 p.m. on February 28, the earth cracked, trembled and shook. I live in California, so I mean this literally. The Upland Earthquake registered 5.5 on the Richter scale across town in Pasadena as the phone rang in the Wapner household. Dr. Gray called to say that I was wiggling my toes, and Joe could come to see me. Sarah and my sister Berty wondered if it had taken an earthquake to awake me.

Things eased a bit at home.

Joe walked into my room. I was lying flat on my back, with a tube in my throat. I couldn't talk. I was staring straight up to the ceiling.

"All I can see are your eyes, big as saucers," Joe said. "When you get out of here, are we going to have a good time!"

All I could do was blink my eyes. I heard every word Joe said.

Joe told me later, "That's when I knew you were going to be OK. The others didn't know, but I did."

For Joe it was not complete relief, just temporary relief, but he was certain I would survive.

Most of the doctors were not as optimistic.

I have been asked repeatedly if, like other written accounts of death experiences, I ever saw white lights or a long tunnel I was traveling through. No. I was comatose. I saw nothing. I felt nothing. I don't remember anything so dramatic as opening my eyes. I had no memory of anything that had happened to me. Carlos told me later that every patient has amnesia for that period, and I have come to believe that forgetting is a blessing.

I have only two recollections. One was the sensation that someone had fondled my left breast; I recall a pleasurable vaginal surge, as well as an attempt to push away the uninvited hand. Maybe this was a dream or a memory of my breasts being rearranged as they were taped down for surgery. It also could have happened as the mammary artery was being "harvested" to be used in the bypass.

Secondly, I remember my body trembling violently as I was being shocked repeatedly to bring me back to life. Not only does the heart have a violent reaction to the shock, but the entire body shakes. What I can say is that I needed no white lights to remind me that I'm very glad to be alive.

Meanwhile, a battery of specialists was summoned. It was late afternoon on February 28, five days after the heart attack.

The infection Carlos and Bill had feared was showing up: I was running a fever of 102 degrees when a specialist in infectious diseases was called in. I had a complex multi-systems disease and with my decreased circulation and oxygen, my liver and bladder should be watched. He recommended antibiotics and warned about avoiding unnecessary risks of increased drug toxicity, and ordered further testing if I showed no improvement.

Dr. Colin Stokol, a neurologist, came to evaluate me. He asked me to open and close my eyes, follow his requests, gaze to the right or left. I was able to move my facial muscles and made some attempt to talk, although I was still on a respirator and had a tube down my throat. He raised some questions about paralysis in my extremities. My limbs were weak and flabby, and he could not determine whether I was able to perceive sensation or a pinch. I could barely squeeze with my right or left hand or push down my right or left leg. I used my arms and legs very little.

My attention span was brief; my gaze slow and incomplete; I was dull and inattentive; however, he had no doubt that I responded and paid attention to him. All of this testing tired and agitated me. If I hadn't had the tube in my mouth, I would have told him to go away and leave me alone. What I didn't know was that he found it very difficult to determine whether I could actually see. To his threatening attempts—he put his finger almost into my eye, waved his hand across my face—I made no response whatsoever.

He thought I might have cortical blindness. He later explained to me "If your eyes fail, then you have ocular blindness, but if you have an injury to the part of the brain that concerns vision, you have what is called 'cortical blindness' because the eyes may work just fine, but if the impulses are not properly handled in the brain, then you have just a blank. You may have normal eyes, and you could still even look at a thing and not see it. You may seem to look a person in the eye and not see him."

By the next day, I was more alert, able to follow objects, but it was too early to assess my memory or vision. I distinctly remember his standing at the foot of my bed holding both his arms upraised with his index and middle fingers spread to a "V." It was one of my most hated memories of Richard Nixon, in his imitation of Winston Churchill's victory sign. To me, it was ludicrous. I didn't know where I'd been, or what had happened to me.

"How many fingers? How many fingers?" he asked. I thought he was nuts.

At the time there was no way to know whether I would be blind, or have any paralysis. Dr. Stokol said. They did not want to move me for a brain scan because they were worried that something would happen.

For him, the question was whether I had already suffered a stroke when I went through my crisis, and there was no simple way for him to tell. What was encouraging was that I would occasionally move all of my limbs, but most times he would pick up one of my legs, and it would flop down like dead weight.

There are no clear records of how long it took for me to be truly "with it," but every day I was climbing the ladder of recovery.

What I hadn't known was that every member of my family and the entire medical team was concerned about blindness, brain damage, paralysis. I had no clues; every time they visited me, my family managed to put on cheerful faces of optimism and encouragement in spite of all they knew.

I knew none of these specifics. I was intensely restless and was sedated to calm me down. I was biting on the hated tube, trying every way I knew how to get it out. I was in severe body pain, still somewhat restrained, although John Bussell preferred to keep me calm with drugs rather than restraints. My body was badly distended, including my ten fingers which were swollen like sausages so no space remained between them. I was purple from the tips of my fingers to my shoulder, the only parts of my body I could see. The nurses were trying to give me a sense of reality, tell me what had happened, how sick

I was, to gently massage my body and put pillow supports all around me to ease the pain and to reassure me. I would be agitated in the morning, calm at night.

A constant admonition to post-surgical patients from their nurses is to cough to get the lungs clear and the mucous flowing. Since I ached all over, they, in their love, wisdom and creativity, devised a method to help me: they folded and folded a flannel sheet into a pillow-size shape, taped it together, drew a large heart with the word, "Mickey" in the center with a bright blue permanent marker and told me to hold it close to my chest as I coughed. Who wouldn't respond to such encouragement? Today the pillow is one of my treasured possessions. A number of major heart hospitals stock a variety of pillows for patients to hug just for this purpose, but mine was handmade, just for me. At this point the tender loving care was helping as much as the medicine. I was improving.

Carlos made plans to remove me from the intra-aortic balloon pump.

So I was going back into surgery for the third (or fourth) time. On March 2, I was returned to the operating room; put under general anesthesia, the staples were removed from my leg, the incision reopened, and the intra-aortic balloon pump that had helped keep my heart beating since the night of the crisis was removed. The hole in my femoral artery was repaired. Again I was sewn up in layers and stapled back together.

It's hard to believe that I was in the operating room for almost a whole day. After that my heart seemed to be functioning relatively well without the support.

Of course, I was still in CSICU, being given dozens of medicines and tests, my body still ridden with pain. I bled, I ran fevers, I suffered great pain and difficulty in coughing, was put back and forth on nitroglycerin drips. My chest and leg incisions, opened and shut so many times, still hurt. And, my breasts were unbearably sore.

But at last the blessed day arrived—they removed the tube from my throat. It didn't matter that I was sore and raw inside, I could talk! It didn't matter that I was tired and my arms and legs felt flabby and weak. By then the doctors showed me a comfortable level of optimism. Carlos said I had made a remarkable recovery; Dr. Stokol found me oriented, remembering two to three objects easily in two minutes, speech clear and my visual acuity improving; Dr. Marcus was optimistic as to the ultimate outcome.

During the nights and days in CSICU, there was a tiresome procession of technicians to take blood, to take electrocardiograms, to take blood pressure, to give inhalation therapy. One night a young man wearing a yarmulke (religious skull cap) came in to give me inhalation therapy.

In between his efforts to give me breathing therapy, I pursued my own agenda. I asked if he would like to come to our house for Sabbath dinner to meet my daughter after I got out of the hospital

"I'm a little shy," he said.

"So is she," I replied, sensing a perfect match in the making.

When I told Fred the story, he decided I must be out of the woods if I could turn my attention to match-making in the middle of the night.

But Carlos noted a continuing infection and a very low blood count. An order was issued for a blood transfusion and a call was put out for blood donors. My son Fred, my brother Bernie, and my friend Frank Zolin, the Executive Officer of the Los Angeles County Superior Court, came to give blood. Luckily, I never needed it.

I was in a post-operative haze, but the thought that Fred and Bernie and Frank would give me the most precious of all gifts, life's blood, gave me comfort, and nothing less than spiritual support. I have since heard blood transfusion recipients marvel at "your blood being in my veins."

I was still weak and fatigued. Tests revealed evidence of pericardial rub from Carlos' squeezing my heart during resuscitation attempts, feeling like two pieces of leather that had been rubbed together. My right ventricle was not working as well as it should have been, and there was also fluid in the sac around the heart. So I wasn't out of danger yet.

On March 6th I was moved by wheelchair out of CSICU to a monitored room. It was the happiest ride I could remember.

But immediately afterwards I was flooded with mixed emotions: from joy to despair, from optimism to fear, from hope to total dependence.

Now I could attempt to read my own mail and receive an avalanche of gifts and the most magnificent plants and flowers I had ever seen. With every letter I cried, with every gift I was overcome with emotion. Soon the room filled to overflowing. I could not believe the expressions of love arriving through my hospital room door and through the atmosphere. It seemed almost selfish to keep all the flowers for myself, so I asked a patient-relations staffer to take pictures, and kept each of them in my room for at least two days before sending them off to the four corners of the hospital where other patients lay without cheer or the attention I received. I still have the pictures and the notes.

The next few days brought more tests and movement toward recovery. Carlos removed the pacing wires and the staples in my chest; he told me I was stable and making a remarkable recovery. I was recovering from the cardiac rub. I was up and about, I had no infection. I could remember two to four objects I had been shown a week ago. I could read small print. All the consultants were off the case. I was never sorry to see any specialist leave; I had Bill, Carlos, and Harold Marcus, my first team, the men I was closest to and whose daily visits were reassuring, cheering and healing through the affection and care they gave me.

Thirteen days after my heart attack I started on cardiac rehabilitation, exercises in bed, and walks in the halls of Cedars-Sinai, always with an attendant. Day by day I increased the distance and stepped up the pace. In some hospitals, the distances are marked off on the corridors, but not here. One day a visiting friend and I were so busy walking and talking that we found ourselves across the hospital in the South Tower Building. Still every bone in my body hurt and I had no idea how long pain would remain my companion.

My next move, to an unmonitored room, was the first step to discharge, and this threw me into a wild panic. The thought of being unmonitored left me feeling vulnerable.

On the day of the move, a nurse told me I would be moving before noon. I waited and waited, panic rising as each hour passed. If I had to move, I wanted to get on with it. Finally, after dinner, I was disconnected from my monitors and moved.

Bernie and Nancy arrived just as I was settled into my new room, and they tried to distract me, change the subject, comfort me. Very soon, Harold Marcus came into my room, unfolded his large, lanky frame into a bedside chair, opened his chart onto his crossed legs and said, "I heard you were pissed."

I burst out laughing.

This wonderful man had found the right tempo and language to ease me. He was sensitive to my anxiety and prescribed a mild sedative. I remained in that room for two days. The night before I left the hospital, a handsome young man came into my room to visit, sat on the window ledge with the night sky back lighting his frame, still wearing his surgical scrub clothes, cap and all. I had had so many teams of interns, residents, cardiologists, cardiac surgeons and fellows visiting during those weeks, I could not recognize him until he took off his cap and let his sandy brown hair fall onto his forehead.

"Don't you remember me, Mickey? I'm John Bussell," he said.

I had not seen him since we spoke the night of surgery.

What I hadn't realized was that John had been the first one to see me move as I was coming out of the coma, and that he had been checking on me regularly during those first days. He describes himself as a low-profile character, so as soon as he felt I was safely on my own, he withdrew to his duties in the operating room.

We moved the flowers off the window seat and sat together talking. I was crying again.

"I'd begun to feel guilty about not seeing you, Mickey," he said, "but I wanted to come to say how glad I am things turned out all right. I knew that you would be asking questions about what happened and pretty soon you'd be putting things together, so I thought I ought to get in here to help you."

John's description of what had happened intensified my sense of astonishment and brought on low sobs, mingled with an outpouring of gratitude for which there are still no adequate words.

"Don't you remember what you said to me?" John said.

At that moment I felt fuzzy, confused. "No, I'm afraid I've forgotten," I said, "Was it something about politics?"

"I gave you that thumbs up sign, and you told me not to do that, it was bad luck, that it was the last thing you saw Robert Kennedy do before he was shot. I couldn't let you go, give up on you after what you said to me that night as we went into surgery. I'm not glad for what happened to you, Mickey, but I want to thank you. We were able to learn a lot from the work we did on you."

I began to shiver and reach for a blanket. His modesty and understanding of my fragile emotional state on that night limited our conversation. Tears of gratitude ran down my cheeks. John put a reassuring arm around my shoulder and promised we would talk to each other soon.

By now I knew a great deal about my case, and that John and Carlos had saved my life. A lot had happened to me physically, emotionally, psychologically and spiritually. Full of gratitude and full of fear and anxiety about my recovery, I slept the last night at a hospital I had grown to love.

Healing is a matter of time, but it is sometimes also a matter of opportunity. HIPPOCRATES

5. looking for answers

I am as willing to accept the spectrum of opinions from my doctors as to what went wrong after surgery, as I am willing to accept that they cannot tell me what caused my heart attack; I can accept that they do not know everything; they are the first to admit it. But what happened to me? During the few days I was struggling back to life, I experienced a wild swing of emotions.

What I tried to show the nurses, my family and closest friends was optimism, cooperation and good humor. What I felt was fear and depression, coupled with wonder and awe. As I lay in the bed, swollen and in intense pain, I remember the first thing I said to Joe: "I don't know what I'm going to do with the rest of my life, but I'm not going to take any shit from anyone." I had already begun to suspect that stress had played a role in my heart attack.

When I first came out of the coma, I didn't know of the cardiac arrest crisis, of the moments I spent on both sides of death's door. All I remembered was that I had said goodbye to Joe and Leah and Bill as I was wheeled into bypass surgery, and I supposed this was the normal way to be waking up. But the parade of specialists and my growing strength made me aware that something very special had happened to me.

Over and over again I heard the word "miracle;" Bill Molle, who was not given to hyperbole, called me a Miracle Woman.

When they finally pulled out the hated tube and I was finished with the four trips to the operating room and its attendant anesthesia, I began to separate myself into two parts: one was the patient in the bed; the other was the recovering self, separate from the patient, looking in on her as if the health crisis had happened to her, not to me. This perception happened so early on that I described it as the nearest thing I'd had to an out-of-body experience. Frequently, when I awakened, I would feel myself separated from that pain-racked, curled-up, swollen patient in the bed—she, shivering with fear, I, smiling toward the future. Perhaps it was denial. The "strong, real Mickey" had separated from the "weak, sick Mickey." After all, the "real Mickey" never gets sick; whatever had happened couldn't have happened to her. Maybe the "strong, real Mickey" could just fly out of there, go home and leave behind the weak half, the imposter. At that moment, I think my head was recovering faster than my body, although there were times later when I was out of sync the other way around—my body recovering and my mind lagging behind. I developed what I called a writerly interest in my own case.

The writer in me was immediately curious, insatiable about the facts, about this patient lying in bed recovering. At the same time I developed a childlike interest in hearing a repitition of the events, very much like, "Tell me the story about my growing up again, mommy." Part of it was that I was not holding thoughts very well; part of it was a budding awareness of what had really happened to me. I was encountering the reality that my doctors, my family, my friends had known for many days—doubts that I would recover at all. That Cedars-Sinai is a teaching hospital was helpful; as the surgeons made rounds with the cardiologists, fellows and residents, the story was told again and again. Slowly it sank in. From Joe's twice daily visits, and his tender, healing care I learned of the vigil, the hundreds of inquiries about my health, the rallying of friends to his side, the outpouring of concern. From my children's faces I saw fear and anxiety turning to hope as I healed. From the avalanche of flowers and gifts I learned that my life had a connectedness, a continuity from childhood to my survival day, that link had not been broken, as I had believed before.

I had survived. And now I was going home to heal.

I witnessed a graceful medical ballet with each actor performing the movement required to complete the task at hand...

6. witnessing bypass surgery

From the time I was in the hospital—even as I split into two personalities and then recovered—my curiosity propelled me to ask Carlos and John for permission to witness bypass surgery. Whether it was to humor me or not, I don't know, but they both agreed, and as we got to know each other during my crisis and recovery, I think they knew I was serious. First I had to get permission from Dr. Jack Matloff, head of the Cardiothoracic Surgery Unit; he agreed. Then I had to get permission from the hospital administration. By the time my request was granted—eighteen months after my heart attack—I went back to Cedars-Sinai to fill in a missing link in my research.

This was my chance to answer questions that I had stored away for a long time. What did the operating room look like? What was the cast of characters involved in the surgery? What was the tempo in the operating room, the interaction between surgeon and staff? How did Carlos direct the surgery? How many tubes was I hooked up to? Where did all those scars on my body come from? How did they cut through my skin, open the rib cage, take the vein and mammary artery? And how did they connect it to my heart? Exactly what is the heart-lung machine? Perhaps witnessing this surgery would link me with my own.

Bill Molle, whose friendship and doctoring have a blurry borderline, accompanied me, mostly to see to my welfare. I had assured everyone, doctors, hospital authorities and my family, that I was not a squeamish person. I expected to handle the surgery well. I had anticipated that the patient could die in surgery and I would have to deal with that; and that if I did get nervous, I would leave the operating room. But Bill didn't want to take any chances with me.

Carlos greeted us warmly and introduced me to Patsy, the head nurse, and to Arnold Friedman, the anesthesiologist. What I didn't realize until I studied my hospital records later, was that Arnie Friedman had been the anesthesiologist when the intra-aortic balloon pump was removed from my leg. It seemed as if every member of that department had had a role in my case.

Patsy took me to the crowded women's locker room, gave me blue scrubs, coverings for my head and shoes, and took me to Carlos at the scrubbing trough. He introduced me to the perfusionist, whose role I began to appreciate and understand as the morning wore on. Arnie Friedman took charge of me and ushered me into the operating room. On the way there I walked through a supply room full of paraphernalia needed for surgeries, past the cramped nurse's lounge filled with nurses laughing and talking, either just off a late night emergency case, or waiting for morning cases. My excitement mounted as I went behind the scenes. As a lay person, I knew I had been granted a rare privilege, and I was determined to learn as much as possible and yet maintain a sense of detachment.

The Operating Room

The operating room is a large, white, rectangular room. Not as imposing as I had expected. As I walked in I heard a loud symphony on the stereo system. I had often wondered when Carlos had time to listen to Mozart, and now I knew; he listens when he operates. I have been told that Dr. Michael DeBakey, of the Baylor College of Medicine in Houston, operates listening to country western music.

A long, rectangular table containing the instruments covered in sterile towels stood away from the far wall. The surgery table was in the center of the room, a small instrument table across from it, the heart-lung machine behind the surgeon.

A totally naked, fully anesthetized, inert 79-year-old woman lay strapped on the operating table. She was a small woman in fine shape, excellent body and muscle tone, pale skin. At first I was startled by the total impersonality of the situation. She might have been a cadaver. To me she was an exposed piece of meat, no dignity whatsoever, not even the courtesy of a cover. That would come later. But as the morning wore on, I began to understand that courtesy is not a part of this procedure; the patient had to be totally disrobed to prepare the body sterilely. To the surgeon and anesthesiologist, to all of the surgical team, it is a human body with no sexual character, no age, no color, no gender, no emotional involvement. Total objectivity.

Unlike my case, hers was elective surgery. Both surgeon and anesthesiologist had had time to see her the night before, take her history, do a physical examination and explain the procedure to her and her family in order to relieve anxiety. Usually a patient is premedicated at that time. What I saw was a patient completely anesthetized, hooked up and ready for surgery, monitors clearly functioning. However, in emergencies like mine, there is no time for premedication, no time for explanations to relieve anxiety; all anesthesiology is done in the operating room.

Arnie explained what he had done. First, he put an intravenous line into a vein, principally to give medications and blood products, whether red blood cells, platelets, fresh or frozen plasma, depending on need or bleeding; after that a catheter was inserted into an artery for measuring blood pressure from heart beat to heart beat. Because things happen very rapidly, this catheter also enables them to give medicine to prevent an excessively high, or a significant drop, in blood pressure. The third catheter is inserted through a vein in the neck, floated through the right side of the heart. From this catheter they get measurements that allow them to determine how much fluid a patient can have safely and what kind of drugs are needed. It also allows them to monitor the electrocardiogram and the muscular function of the heart, to take blood samples, to determine how well the patient is oxygenating (whether he/she needs more or less oxygen), or to do certain manipulations to expand the lungs. The anesthetic is introduced through one of the catheters. Only after the patient is completely asleep the endotracheal tube is put in the mouth, down into the bronchial tree, to breathe for the patient. As I remembered my crisis, I knew it was lucky for me that these catheters remained in place after surgery so they could be quickly hooked up again for my emergency post-bypass surgery.

Personnel

The cast of characters in the operating room are the surgeon, assistant surgeon, physician's assistant, the scrub nurse, who is scrubbed sterile, handing instruments to the surgeon, the circulating nurse, who breaks open the sterile packages and drops instruments on the table for the surgeon, the perfusionist, who runs the heart-lung machine, the anesthesiologist, and the anesthesia technician, who makes sure all the electronic monitoring equipment is working and who can repair them if needed. Until I saw them work together, I could not fully appreciate the concept of team medicine.

I stood in the anesthesiologist's station, no more than three feet wide and five feet deep, immediately behind the head of the patient on the operating table. Metal poles at each end of this table held bags of fluid. Everything Arnie needed was within reach. Behind him was another tray where he could retrieve additional anesthesia or instruments as needed. There were three monitors, one almost at eye level that Carlos could see from his position, another across the table for the assistant surgeon, so they have instantaneous and continuous monitoring, and another, independent of the other two, for Arnie to register his calculations for measurements that allow him to decide on medications and dosages.

Preparing the Patient

Carlos came into the operating room with a mask covering his beard, hat over his head, surgical glasses on his face. It was as if I saw him for the first time. The scrub nurse helped him into his sterile robe and surgical gloves. Soon I would see what I had come for.

He stood at the right side of the patient, the physician's assistant to his right by the patient's leg. He faced Patsy, the circulating nurse, and the assistant surgeon across from the patient.

Just before Carlos began surgery, I went out to the nurses supply station to get an additional scrub blouse. I had been so preoccupied that I hardly breathed and didn't realize how cold I was.

Carlos and the physician's assistant and the nurse began to prepare the patient. Her body had already been cleansed and swabbed with iodine for cleanliness and sterility. She lay on a blue sheet, gathered up all around to make a drainage trough. Carlos unwrapped the package of sterile bydrape, a plastic, iodine coated adhesive sheeting, and Patsy helped him draw it firmly across the body of the patient. It was as if they had completely enveloped her already scrubbed body in Saran wrap. The purpose was for continuous sterilization of the body as the surgery proceeded. With a black marker they drew a line on both her legs to indicate the probable locale for the incision to harvest the saphenous vein from the leg. They draped her with small blue cloths, pushing towels into her crotch, over her left leg, leaving her right leg exposed, covering her arms and her head. Then they dropped the curtain almost to her chin line so that her head was separated from the other part of her body. The curtain hung right in front of me between the operating table and the anesthesiologist's station.

They raised the poles and curtain up to about six feet, and I was afraid I wouldn't be able to see, but Arnie placed two stacked stools against the table for me to stand on and watch. He asked me if I had any questions; to ask anything I wanted. But I was prepared. For my own notes and questions, I had put a notebook and pen in my pocket, and off and on during the surgery, I jotted questions down. As the surgery proceeded, Arnie drew me a picture of what to expect, explained every cut and stitch throughout the operation.

The Heart-Lung Machine

Somehow, without knowing why, I had a cartoonist's perception of the heart-lung machine shaped like a combined heart and lung. (When I actually saw it, I thought if someone pressed a button, it would start to play oom-pah-pah like an old-fashioned calliope.) When I was told I had been on the machine for only a relatively short time, it meant nothing to me. What I saw that day was a big gleaming white and stainless steel sophisticated and complex machine with tubes and valves and gauges that occupies a large space and an important role in the operation. Had this machine not been invented, this surgery would not be possible. Had the technology not been in place, nothing could have happened. The machine acts as a substitute for the patient's circulation system. About ninety-nine percent of the blood is drained from the body through a tube. The blood is passed through a complex filter that acts as a substitute lung and purification system; the machine takes the blood, separates it, moves it from chamber to chamber and recirculates it in a series of tubes that somewhat approaches the system of blood circulation in the body.

I saw the blood of the patient drain from her own circulatory system and move to the machine. As the surgery progressed, I saw the pump in the chest showing the simulated heart beat and lung function. When the pump motion decreases, the heart beat diminishes. The blood is being cooled as it flows through the system.

I had the antiquated idea that I had been cooled down by being placed on an ice mattress, never any sense of the blood being drained away, cooled, recirculated, no appreciation of the complexity of the machine and its multiple functions. Most doctors agreed that it was because my body—my heart and my brain—had been cooled down to such a low temperature that I survived the cardiac arrest and subsequent crisis. Neither organ requires much oxygen at a low temperature. One major reason I survived, very much like stories about kids "drowning," falling into freezing lakes, being rescued and surviving, was because of the big machine at one side of the operating room.

THE SURGERY

Carlos made the first cut through the plastic sheeting and first and second layers of skin with a fine scalpel. I smelled a faint order of burnt skin. He cut quickly and cleanly through the sternum (the breast bone) with a tiny mechanized saw. It was not as disagreeable to watch as I had anticipated. As he worked, he sponged so that very little blood was apparent. When the rib cage was completely severed, they took a clamp and pushed and cranked the sternum apart, then cranked it apart some more, and spread an opening to reveal the field for the operation.

As they pushed and cranked those ribs apart, my hand reached instinctively for my chest; at that moment, I understood why my ribs hurt, why my breasts had hurt so much for such a long time. My rib cage had been opened twice within a few hours. And pushed, and cranked apart. And pushed, and cranked back together. And pushed and cranked apart and pushed and cranked back together another time.

Carlos cut through the pericardial sac. Arnie leaned over my shoulder and described what lay exposed before my eyes — the lung, gray and pinkish, with tiny black lines; the heart, the branching arteries, the fat around the heart, the pericardium sac, the left descending artery that was to be bypassed, just like mine. We stepped back to Arnie's table as he drew a picture of what would come next.

Sponging as he went, Carlos' long fingers explored her heart. Before he went in, he had not known how many bypasses would be needed or whether an aortic valve needed replacement, but he decided the leakage from the aorta had been caused by the fistula they had seen on the X-ray. Only three bypasses. Meanwhile, the physician's assistant cut through the black line on the leg and exposed the saphenous vein.

At that moment the blood pressure dropped. Carlos, whose voice had been barely audible, raised his voice and said "I need another surgeon and I need him right now." He asked why the blood pressure was dropping and ordered drugs to stabilize the condition. Arnie reached through my legs to insert the drugs into the proper container. I could see the blood pressure stabilize on the monitor.

The only moment that broke the apparent calm was when the nurse got on the phone and quite agitatedly asked someone to please get Dr. so and so—and get him there right now. Carlos, working very quickly, would need the vein before the veins would be ready for his use. The arriving surgeon helped the physician's assistant remove the vein. They stretched it out on the side table, examined it, tied off any imperfections and cut it into pieces, put them in a container of liquid to be ready for Carlos.

BYPASS

The smell of burned flesh permeated the room as Carlos cauterized to stanch the flow of blood as he cut. He took the mammary artery, cut it off at one end, inserted it into the heart and stitched it into place to bypass the damaged artery. The veins were fished out of the bottle, sewn at two ends like a bridge over the remaining damaged arteries. I watched Carlos sew with the tiniest hook-shaped needle, working by feel and skill. Every stitch precise, perfect.

Now I knew what a bypass was. The fresh, undamaged mammary artery and saphenous veins were sewn at each end and around the blocked portions of the arteries, making a little loop not more than an inch in length to bypass around the blockage, leaving the blocked portion in place. Now the blood had fresh, open channels to flow through. I saw those loops with my own eyes. I suppose I might have known about this had I come in for elective surgery, read some books, asked more questions, or read more carefully the booklet Cedars-Sinai gave to me, but I didn't get the picture until it was right before me.

As Carlos worked, he asked for more ice chips and water to be poured directly into the sac to keep things cold. He poured, the nurse poured and siphoned out the extra liquid. The excess trickled into the drainage trough around the operating table sheets.

The bypasses completed, the blood was returned from the machine to the patient's body. Her heart fluttered, began to beat on its own. The lung began to move on its own, the pump slowed and flattened as the lungs took over. Just below the rib cage line, they punched drains from the pericardium to the outside of her body and tied the fine stitching off with colored silk threads. I remembered the bright red, green, blue, and yellow tassels dangling under my breasts, as well as "X" scars left behind. As Carlos pushed the drains through, I again felt for my chest and understood the pain during recovery.

Carlos called the physician's assistant to help him close. He laced a heavy metal wire through one side of the rib cage and across into the other. Another wire, in one side, across to the other. Another, and another, until about eight heavy metal wires spanned the opening. Then he and his assistant, each pulling against the other, pulled the rib cage back together, assisted again by the crank. They wound them off and twisted them with an implement which had been used to hold the wire. I suppose it is the end of those wires that I feel as little balls I can roll with my fingers, little bumps on my chest, just underneath the incision line. He finished stitching the two layers of skin together, clamped the final layer of chest and leg incisions together.

And that was it. Here was a 79-year-old woman given a second chance at life.

Toward Recovery

These five hours went by almost in the blink of an eye. I had stood no more than three feet from Carlos, watching a procedure he had performed on me. No more mystery about the surgery. Exhilarated and awe-struck, I was startled when Carlos took the last stitch, looked up at me and asked if I wanted to accompany the patient to the Cardiac Surgery Intensive

Care Unit. I watched as the nurses came in from intensive care, pulled away the bloody towels that surrounded her, took off the tape that had covered her eyes, and covered her with warm flannel sheets before transferring her from the operating table to her new bed. We set off for CSICU. For a few minutes it seemed like a funeral, the nurses as pall bearers, Arnie as the clergyman accompanying the body, and I as the mourner, following the cortege.

But not before I noticed the paddles they had used to shock my heart, trying to get me to come back. Just as I had done creating a cartoon image in my mind about the heart-lung machine, I somehow had envisioned this shocking device as an old-fashioned permanent wave machine, with wires and clamps hanging down carrying electric current to the heart. Instead, I saw benign, black plastic paddles, twelve inches long, two inches in diameter. Nothing antiquated or barbarian. A modern machine designed for use in an emergency, as needed.

I had witnessed a professional, organized effort, no extraneous act or conversation and no mistakes that I could see, with respect between surgeon and his team. A peaceful medical ballet with each actor performing the movement required to complete the particular task at hand, no more, no less. So this was what had happened to me. The sense of awe about my crisis was rekindled.

While I thought I had been thoroughly absorbed in the drama in the operating room, thoughts of my own surgery crept in during the entire time. But nowhere did the association become as strong as when we moved from the controlled environment of the operating room to the CSICU. As her tapes and bloody sponges were removed, and her small body covered in a warm sheet, I watched the "rehumanization" of the patient.

Arnie accompanied the patient back to the room, and I listened as he transferred the information from operating room to recovery and engaged in informal banter with the nurse and cardiologist who would be in charge of the patient during this initial phase of recovery. It was at this moment that I appreciated how important the partnership between John and Carlos, between surgeon and anesthesiologist had been. I was shocked at the change between the mood in the operating room and the rather loud voices joking about procedures, perhaps covering the stress of their responsibility in CSICU. I knew it was only within minutes of my arrival in this room that my trouble had begun.

Suddenly I began to shiver, and decided I had seen enough. It was time to leave. I took off my scrub clothes, put on my street clothes and went to say good-bye to Carlos. It was a perfunctory farewell, and I walked out of his office and out of Cedars-Sinai. The surgery had been the easiest part. As I thought of that woman upstairs, I knew that it was during this moment after my surgery that all hell had broken loose and I had gone on the critical list. Fear and dread had me shaking all the way home.

Epidemiologic studies show that some form of stress can be a trigger in perhaps half of heart attacks.   Dr. Noel Bairey Merz

7. stress: long term

I might never know how or why I survived my post surgery crisis, but I wanted to see if I could find out what caused my heart attack. Could it have been stress? Before drawing that conclusion, I explored my medical history over the past thirty years.

There are five notations on my chart worth repeating.

On November 18, 1974: Has been jogging this a.m. Chest burning... and this has persisted.

October 29, 1982: Chest pains and fatigue. Recently under much stress (Sarah and at work). b.p. 140/80

April 12, 1984: Severe pain in low back after emotional upset. Localized. b.p. 130/80.

July 19, 1988: Palpitations lately. Four times past couple of months. b.p. 120/78. (I was given a bottle of pills to take if palpitations reoccurred.)

These symptoms in a man would have prompted a stress test. I was a woman, and consequently a stress test was not ordered.

Generally my lifestyle could be described as moderate. My cholesterol hovered around the 200 mark, sometimes up to 216, sometimes down to 179. My blood pressure was normal. I never smoked. I did not have diabetes. I drank socially, but rarely to excess. There was no history of heart disease in my family. My exercise regimen was irregular, but over the past fifteen years I had become a fairly steady walker. Since the onset of menopause, I had been on hormone replacement therapy (premarin and provera).

Most of the time I thought I was overweight, a yo-yoing up and down by ten pounds or less, so in my early years I was frequently on a diet to lose weight. I fed my family the recommended balanced diet of the day: meat, cheese, dairy products, along with fruits and vegetables. As new nutritional guidelines were developed, I modified our family's diet accordingly. At the same time, when I was upset I would stuff myself or go on eating binges. I called it my "hand-to-mouth" disease.

My behavior, however, was not moderate. I was a high energy, hard-driving woman, juggling my family, work and social responsibilities, always trying to cram one more activity into a day. On vacation, I would try to jam as much as I could into a day. I remember dragging Joe to the Washington Zoo at dusk because I wanted to see the pandas.

Much of the time I felt my life was dictated from the outside, not by my choices. Frustration, hurt and anger penetrated my thin skin. But need for approval had me putting on a good face, holding in, reigning in my tension. Even resting, I conducted my life in high gear. I couldn't turn my brain off. I didn't know I was setting myself up for trouble down the line.

To learn more about stress, specifically how it relates to heart disease, I spoke to Dr. C. Noel Bairey Merz, medical director of the Preventive and Rehabilitation Cardiac Center of Cedars-Sinai Medical Center and an assistant clinical professor of medicine at the UCLA School of Medicine. She drew me a small diagram.

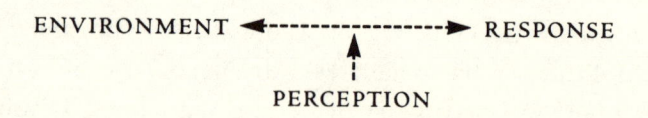

ENVIRONMENT ◄--------------► RESPONSE
▲
│
PERCEPTION

Environment (your life and its circumstances), your perception of it, and your response to it are three important components to stress. Many people have a lot of environmental stress and personally perceive it as stressful, yet their bodies don't react to it—their brain does. This protective mechanism, a good separation between brain and body, doesn't hurt their heart. By contrast, there are a number of people who take the environmental stress, perceive it as stressful, and their physiology—the way their heart functions, and their blood pressure goes up, and the way their vessels constrict their response turns this into something that can hurt their heart.

Dr. Dean Ornish concurs: *"Between the environment and our reactions to it are our perceptions.* Our perceptions determine how we react to a situation and whether or not that reaction is going to be harmful to us."

As I struggled to understand how I dealt with my anger, I wondered if it would have been better to blurt it out rather than suppress it as I did. Carol Tavris, in her book, "Anger: The Misunderstood Emotion," writes that "expressing anger makes you angrier." Her research shows that ventilating anger usually does more harm than good.

Stress, as Dr. Bairey Merz defines it, operates on many levels. First, stress probably contributes to atherosclerosis, plaques. Next, stress can turn the plaques into a clinical event. And finally, stress appears to trigger heart attacks and cardiac deaths.

"We have mounting evidence at this time that stress in humans is a good trigger ischemia, an early warning sign of a heart attack," she said. "Epidemiologic studies show that some form of stress can be a trigger in perhaps half of heart attacks."

I asked Dr. Bairey Merz if there was any way to alter the formation of plaque caused by stress.

"We need to knock out only one factor of the environment/response/perception triangle," she said,

"Studies have shown a fifty percent reduction in recurrent

heart disease deaths if any of these learned behaviors can be modified. There are ways to alter behaviors, but it requires hard work. But first the patient has to admit to himself or herself that there is a problem. Preventive cardiology consists of behavioral changes in diet, exercise, response to stress, life style and a change in the way a person looks at life.

"In general, it doesn't look like getting angry helps you," Dr. Bairey Merz said. "We used to think, 'Oh it's because they keep it all in.' That's why they got heart disease. They're very angry, but they keep it all in, and it hurts their heart.

"It looks like shouting doesn't help either. The problem is being angry." she said, "but there are behavioral ways you can help yourself to not become angry so often, but they involve a whole different way of looking at life."

An increasing body of research is being conducted into stress as one of the components of heart disease. Stress had been given little credence because it was difficult to quantify stress in humans; most research had been done on animals. And subsequently most human research was done on males.

Dr. Hans Selye's animal research, done in 1926 and refined in 1956, demonstrated that the body "pays a price for the way it responds to stress."

Then came Drs. Meyer Friedman and Ray Rosenman's research which established that "Type A behavior—ambitious, aggressive, competitive, hostile feelings and behavior—is linked specifically to coronary heart disease in humans."

But Type A behavior has been called into question recently by a number of researchers, among them Dr. Redford Williams, Director of Behavioral Research at Duke University Medical Center.

Williams and his colleagues concluded that anger and hostility are the most health-damaging personality traits of type A behavior.

Up to now—and here's the joker again—all this research has been done on men. We don't know if a woman can have a

Type A personality and what it might mean to her heart. Women have not been studied (re: stress) and are only now beginning to be studied where heart disease is concerned.

As for me and my immoderate behavior, did I ever put my feet up when the pressure was on? Did I ever remove myself from the arena of stress? Did I ever take a long, slow bath instead of a quick shower? I don't remember ever doing so.

Dr. Robert S. Eliot, of the Institute of Stress medicine, Denver, Colorado, was a cardiovascular consultant to the U.S. Government at Cape Canaveral in 1967, when he investigated the alarming rate at which young aerospace workers were dropping dead. While the physical and laboratory exams of engineers showed no unusual levels of the standard coronary risk factors, his studies showed that stress from the knowledge and fear of firing caused high levels of anxiety and depression, and a universal, pervasive feeling of hopelessness and helplessness. Their lifestyle, their reaction to their environment, caused acute stress.

Analysis of autopsies of those workers who had dropped dead without warning showed that adrenaline and other stress chemicals had spewed into their bodies with such strength that they had literally ruptured the muscle fibers of their hearts.

More recently, Eliot used well-established scientific methods to measure the physiologic, biochemical, and clinical responses to stress on the cardiovascular system. In the lab, patients were fitted with electrodes and seated in a soundproof room. They were challenged with tasks like mental arithmetic and video games. Critical functions, including heart rates and blood pressure were recorded on computers.

Using this tool to establish a crucial link between health and stress, Eliot's team examined their patients' sources of stress and their styles for coping with it in their emotional, behavioral, and cardiovascular responses. Additional evaluations by a psychologist, dietitian, exercise therapist and a medical examination were brought together to create a treatment program.

Dr. Bairey Merz also conducted structured mental tests in the laboratory.

Dr. Lynda Powell, an epidemiologist at the Yale School of Medicine, and her researchers are involved in a study which is trying to determine what women and men who have suffered heart attacks find stressful.

Many of the men respond with traditional Type A behaviors. But the older women manifest their stress through resentment, keeping anger inside without overt manifestations. A Stanford University team found that anxiety, fearfulness, hostility, and anger are psychological traits that predispose people to second heart attacks. While hostility and anger are more harmful to men, anxiety and fearfulness seem to be more harmful to women. Younger women react differently.

I remember coming home from work, (this was when my kids were older) and I couldn't even get inside the house before they were on the steps asking questions. Joe was often just behind them. I was on duty before I could unload my packages or take a deep breath.

In a recent study American working women cite stress as the most significant job related problem they encounter. Nearly three-quarters of women in their 40's who hold professional and management jobs listed stress as their top problem, as did more than two-thirds of single working mothers.

Women face a variety of stresses in the work force, but stress of work is exceedingly difficult to evaluate, especially because of the lack of research on the effect of the workplace on women. Again, the few studies that have been done use methods adapted from studies of working men; and since women rotate in and out of the workplace, it is more difficult to evaluate the workplace, according to Dr. Ellen Hall, an assistant professor of behavioral science and health education at Johns Hopkins University.

While it is known that social isolation is more stressful for women than men, labor studies do not measure the amount and importance of the social support some women gain from their jobs.

And women who try to cross over into non-traditional occupations face special stresses. Until studies are designed which take all these factors into consideration, it will be difficult to evaluate the true effect of outside jobs on women, says Dr. Hall.

Pressure on working women is growing even worse as they are forced to take up second jobs, because they need the money.

Women are socialized to be "pleasers," and as a result they are too often torn between loyalties, divided among husband, children, aging parents, co-workers, and boss.

Women are also socialized to take too much responsibility on themselves, and the unrealistic demands they place on themselves manifests itself as potentially health harming stress.

As I tried to find causes of my heart attack words came back to me, "Under any stress?"

I thought it was fair to examine the kinds of things that have bothered me during my lifetime. That I have lived with them, and learned to function effectively, or to cope, does not tell me how or whether any junk was deposited on my arteries, little by little, over the decades that it took to build up, crack apart and tumble into a troublesome chasm. What were my fears, my anxieties, my frustrations? What made me clam up and control my anger? What made me blast out in fury those times that I lost control? What made me take these things to heart?

So with this august company of experts, how do I have the chutzpah to give my own definition of stress? I looked upon my stress as my reaction to a single event, or an accumulation of events, that make me angry and anxious and that I can't shake off or recover from within a short period. Something I carry with me, unexplored, perhaps like a time bomb, unexploded, ticking away, reminding me that something is disturbing me. Sometimes I can't put my finger on it, sometimes I can, but I can't unload it. I carry it inside. I think most women do.

I asked Dr. Ann Hickey, a cardiologist who writes on women and heart disease, "When does it begin?"

"If you're willing, go all the way back to your early childhood," she said.

I'm willing to make that painful journey if it helps women identify stress in their lives. Stress that leads to illness. Stress that can be prevented.

What, if anything, predestines us for stress?

8. stresses of early life

All lives are stressful, but some of us deal with stress in less successful ways than others. Who was this woman hovering between life and death? And what had brought her to Cedars-Sinai? This apparently most unlikely patient to have a heart attack?

I was born in the first year of my immigrant parents' marriage, in Mercedes, a small Mexican border town in South Texas. They were learning to speak both English and Spanish, opening a small dry goods store and getting to know each other. (We did not learn about the strain of those early days for many years.) So it is no wonder that cooperation became my modus. Even as a baby, I must have sensed the stress they were experiencing, but all they told us about those days was that they worked hard and were happy to be in this country.

I believe stress, and how we cope and adapt to it, is learned at a very early age. If we learn to deal with it we can be healthy; if not, it will haunt us the rest of our lives. But humans are always capable of change. I've changed, even if it took me a lifetime of stress and a life threat to accomplish it.

Later, when I went to school, I experienced and observed that we were in a highly stratified society, albeit in a small Texas border town. There were the Anglos, who looked down on everybody else; a large population of Mexicans who, hundreds of years before, had pioneered and settled the region; and a small odd assortment of others, a couple of Negroes, a gypsy and a few Jews.

We Jews fit in nowhere, yet those of us who were white had the tacit acceptance of the Anglo community. From my earliest memories, I felt the stress of not belonging. But no one socialized across what we now call ethnic lines. I don't know what expectations my parents brought with them, except the hope that freedom would provide opportunity. Having come from highly segregated villages, they probably expected no more. If my parents were hurt by social exclusion, they never talked about it.

I don't remember liking my sister at all, and we did not become friends till we were adults. I felt that my young brothers had privileges and a special place in the family because they were boys. What I do remember were my mother's lectures about loving my sister and brothers. My feelings of frustration were turned inside me as anger. I was a good little girl, I didn't "talk back"; expressing my feelings only led to rebukes and guilt. I believe that this set the pattern for how I coped in my life. (I did, however, slap my sister's face when we were in college in an uncharacteristic outburst of anger.)

I was insanely jealous of my sister, who I believed had a closer relationship with my father. Many years later, after his suicide, we began sharing stories and letters and I discovered that I was right—He did have a warmer, closer relationship with her. His letters to her were caring, somewhat philosophical and filled with narratives and words of advice. To this day, I remember receiving the most perfunctory letters, and the only one I saved is one he wrote on my twenty-first birthday, quite loving and philosophical, but also stiffer and more dutiful than those to my sister.

When I was six years old my mother gave birth at home to my brother Harry. I remember a lot of commotion and being shunted out of the way. Eight days later, throngs of Jews came to the little town from all over the Rio Grande Valley and crowded into our house to observe my brother's *Brit Milah*, ritual circumcision ceremony. I am not sure if I had ever seen a penis before, and I wondered at the jubilation that surrounded the celebration of such a thing.

We had never had so much company, and I was chagrined at the goings-on as my sister and I pushed our way through the legs of the men gathered around my father holding my new baby brother. I heard someone say something about God, and if this was God's idea, I didn't think God was too smart.

What was all this about, I wondered; I didn't ask, and no one told me. I was excluded. On that day, the most special thing in the world, it seemed to me from my three-foot-high sight line, was to be a baby boy and have everyone celebrating your maleness and your penis.

Many years later, when my first son was circumcised at a home ceremony and celebration, I stayed in my bedroom in horror. Even then I couldn't speak up and say, "No, I won't have it here. I won't have it this way." I relived the pain of my childhood. Still piling on the stress and being reminded of early pain. I never talked about it. I held it in. For our second son, I insisted that it be done in the hospital.

I have come a long way in altering my attitude and behavior through many years of studying the Bible, Jewish history and ritual; moreover, I have become an ardent Jewish feminist. I recognize the patriarchal slant of our religion and the toll it has taken on women over centuries. It is as if we didn't exist in our own history. Rather than suffer the pain, I now speak up to correct the exclusion and injustice.

Does the pain you feel as a child go to your heart? Was it stress? Does plaque begin at the age of six? I don't know.

All I ever wanted in those years was to have something I couldn't get: to have my father love me as much as he did my sister. To be a little boy, to have a penis, and to have as much fuss made over me as was made over my brother. To be a Christian like all my best friends at school, or at least to be acknowledged as a Jew and treated as an equal. To fit in. To be like the others.

Mother and I went back to my fortieth high school class reunion, only to be reminded of how things had been. Some of my old Anglo girl friends had had a mother-daughter tea the day before the reunion. Mother and I were not invited. Even forty years later, I felt the sting of exclusion; it was as if Mother and Daddy's social life and my own were being played out again in the same way and in the same place as before. I really never knew if those Anglo families socialized together, but I was sure they did. It was our family as a whole that couldn't seem to make it, that didn't fit in.

This was all played out against the background of the gathering holocaust overseas, Nazi laws of discrimination and exclusion, confiscation of property, systematic persecution, arrest, torture, then murder of Jews all over Europe. In 1937 Mother left Mercedes for Lithuania to try to persuade her parents and brother to come to America, to be saved from a fate my parents knew would befall them. My grandfather thought that America was an irreligious country. A devout, orthodox, observant Jew, he refused.

At the same time, a virulent wave of anti-Semitism ran rampant in the United States during the 1930's and 1940's. Jews were excluded from many social organizations. Clubs and resorts discriminated and would not allow Jews to enter. Many major universities and professional schools had discriminatory admission quotas. Jews knew where they were welcome and where unwelcome. They objected quietly, but nobody made waves. The country was in the grip of the Ku Klux Klan, and the few voices of protest and good-will were drowned out of raucous public demonstrations of hatred.

No one in Mercedes ever said to us, "We're sorry to hear of the Nazis' measures against the Jews." Neither our teachers, our customers, our schoolmates, their families, nor the ministers, ever spoke a kind or understanding word to us.

We were quiet, too.

More and more we gravitated to the other Jewish families in the Rio Grande Valley. It was as if we wanted to shrink back into ourselves, our own group, for protection. There were many German families in our town, most of them friendly, but we weren't sure if they secretly were members of the local Nazi Bunds (pro-Nazi organizations in the United States during the 1930's and 1940's). We didn't know. I was so ambivalent. Wanting to fit in, be like the others, fearing for the safety of my mother's family in Lithuania. At the same time, I began to feel ashamed of my parents' foreign accents, and feeling guilty for it, even as I loved them and admired their energy, resourcefulness and achievements in that little town. I wanted to get away, to try my wings in a bigger place. The University of Texas was it.

College was both more and less than I wanted. I whirled into a dizzying spiral upward, learning, growing, falling in love, moving into a profession: journalism. It was here that I became a political activist. I learned my craft by moving from reporter to feature writer to editor at The Daily Texan, and ended up being elected by the student body as Associate Editor.

For me another definition of stress is wanting and not having. If I had known how to ascertain my wants and needs, to be able to articulate them, I would have been better off; I would not have carried so much frustration—is that a synonym for stress?—like carrying debits and credits forward in a ledger, never losing any account or entry. I was now more ambitious than I realized.

What I had really wanted in 1945 was to be the editor of The Daily Texan, our college newspaper. If I had said to Horace Busby, "I want to be editor, and you be associate editor, and we'll run as a team," it would probably have been more truthful to my feelings. Instead, I said, "You run as editor, I'll run as associate, and we'll run as a team." Even then, at 20 years old, I was bound by conventions. After all, wasn't it a woman's place to stand back, give way to a man?

So it was not without a strong sense of my own talent that I set out to find a job in Los Angeles, unknown, without contacts and in a state that did not value my training and journalism degree from the University of Texas.

Part Two

The leading cause of death for women is heart disease.

9. matters and myths of the heart:
THE GENDER GAP

Heart attacks happen to men. For a variety of reasons, that's what we've always thought. Our disease: breast cancer. Celebrities flood the talk-show circuit discussing it. We hear a steady drumbeat about the importance of mammograms and self-exams. We're given the statistics everyday—women have a one-in-nine lifetime risk of developing breast cancer. We know all the risk factors. We know our family history. We know everything there is to know about this awful disease.

Most of us don't know that heart disease kills six times as many women as breast cancer. That as many women die of heart attacks or other cardiovascular diseases as men. That the one-in-nine figure is recited on cue, pales in comparison to our lifetime risk of succumbing to heart disease: one in two.

Why don't we know?

Part of it is perception. Breast cancer often afflicts young women. Similarly, middle-aged men die of heart attacks; premenopausal women rarely do. (We catch up later.) People pay more attention when disease strikes early.

But the experts, too, have looked at heart disease almost exclusively as a man's problem, despite the fact that women dying of it isn't anything new—since 1920, more American women have died of heart ailments than of any other cause. Still, the American Heart Association's first public conference for women, held in 1964, taught participants how to care for their husbands' hearts. Medical students learning about heart disease were told not to worry about women.

Most tellingly, women have long been left out as subjects of cardiovascular research—or of any other area of medical study, for that matter. Scientists have feared that pre-menopausal women's hormonal cycles might skew test results, or that a woman would unknowingly become pregnant and expose her fetus to an exploratory drug. What's more, most researchers have excluded persons over the age of sixty out of concern that their poorer general health might confound the data. Since women develop heart disease at least a decade after men and are largely protected prior to menopause, this age bias doubles as a gender bias.

The one notable exception to the men-only rule, the Framingham Heart Study, began following 5,000 men and women in the city of Framingham, Massachusetts, in 1948. By the mid 1950's, the Framingham researchers concluded that chest pain was far more likely to predict a heart attack within five years for a man than for a woman. Women, it seemed, were much less affected by heart disease.

There were two problems: first, though chest pain is frequently associated with angina (a symptom of heart disease in which narrowed coronary arteries cause a shortage of oxygen to the heart muscle), later studies found that women with chest pain are three times more likely than men not to have blocked arteries. And second, it turns out that women suffer from angina for much longer than men before having a heart attack. The Framingham women were simply too young. Two-thirds of them were pre-menopausal. Nonetheless, the early results perpetuated the long-held myth.

Even when they acknowledged that women were susceptible, physicians always assumed that the research conducted on men was equally applicable to women. Only very recently, in the face of mounting evidence to the contrary, has the scientific community begun to conclude what, to many, would seem a given: men and women are physiologically distinct, and what we know about one generally doesn't always carry over to the other.

With that admission comes the daunting realization that on many matters related to women and their hearts, we're starting from scratch.

The best strategies for preventing heart disease? We know what works for men; it will take time to discover whether what works for women is the same. Aspirin? Low doses proved helpful in men; we have little data on the drug's impact on women. Estrogen replacement after menopause? You guessed it — this potentially useful therapy, gender-specific as it is, has just begun to be addressed.

Scientists are finally getting on track. At last a fair number of studies have begun looking at how the heart differs in men and women, and at female-specific aspects of coronary disease. The National Institutes of Health — the country's largest underwriter of medical research — has embarked on the Women's Health Initiative, a massive $600 million, 14-year study in which the 140,000 research subjects are all female. But it will take time before this gender gap is closed — and perhaps even longer to change the thinking of millions of Americans, physicians included, who were brought up to think of heart disease as a man's problem

What do we know? During our reproductive years, natural estrogen seems to protect us from heart disease — approximately ninety percent of heart disease deaths among women occur after menopause. When menopause hits, estrogen levels drop and heart disease in women begins a steep climb. By age 67, it is the number one female killer, striking women and men indiscriminately.

Partly because women develop heart disease 10–15 years later in life than men, they fare worse. A woman is twice as likely as a man to die soon after her first heart attack; if she survives, she is more apt to suffer debilitating pain and disability, and more likely to have a second attack.

The fundamental heart-attack cause knows no gender—plaque accumulates and blood clots form along the coronary arteries, restricting the flow of blood to the heart. For men, this process generally begins in their 40's. Women at that age are typically still producing natural estrogen, which raises HDL levels (the "good" cholesterol that rids the body of blood fats) and lowers LDL (the "bad" cholesterol that sticks around as fat, narrowing the arteries).

When the ovaries shut down at menopause, estrogen levels drop and women begin the process that men have already started. One question raised by recent research, though, is whether menopause simply takes away women's natural advantage—their hormones—or if, in fact, the menopausal changes themselves create risks beyond the loss of the estrogen protection. The University of Pittsburgh's Healthy Women Study has found that menopause and the aging process both contribute to a boost in women's LDL cholesterol and fibrinogen, a blood-clotting substance that raises heart-disease risk. So while women clearly have a pre-menopausal advantage, we might also be at a post-menopausal handicap. More research will say for sure.

We know that from their mid-30's to their mid-60's, women are more susceptible than men to the heart-disease risks of hypertension, high levels of blood glucose, and obesity. Women's heart-disease symptoms tend to be more subtle than men's. While a man's pain is often sudden and severe, extending through the chest or left arm, women are more likely to experience a lingering pain accompanied by nausea, dizziness, sweatiness and vomiting. They are also more apt to experience other symptoms without chest pain. And after an attack, women's hearts seem to heal differently.

The wild-card factor is stress. Because it is difficult to measure, we may never know exactly to what extent stress contributes to heart disease, but few question its significance. Anger, for one, stimulates the release of the hormone norepinephrine, which constricts blood vessels at the same time that the heartbeat is accelerating. This elevates the blood pressure, further straining the heart and vessels.

Stressful situations, of course, are defined by the individual. One person's idea of a challenging experience might be another's nightmare; this is one of among the reasons it's difficult to study stress's effect on the heart based on people's reaction to the same event. But of equal interest are the differences in the way individuals process what is stressful to them. One possibility that's been suggested is that a genetic or acquired deficiency explains why some people are less able to adapt to stress than others and makes them more susceptible to the stress-related development of heart disease.

Going even further, Dr. C. Noel Bairey Merz found a gender-based difference in the handling of stress: in post-menopausal women, stressful stimuli raise the blood pressure and heart rate and cause the arteries to squeeze shut.

Is stress a greater risk factor for heart disease in postmenopausal women than in men? This, too, will be something to watch. We don't have the data yet, but finally the studies are being done.

Perhaps the worst manifestation of the heart disease gender gap can be found in diagnosis and treatment. Study upon recent study tell us that at every step—from interpreting and treating symptoms to ordering tests and referring for angioplasty or bypass surgery—women with heart disease are treated less aggressively than men.

A psychotherapist friend asked a few of her clients two questions: 1. How do you define stress? and 2. How do you experience it physically? Their replies:

Paul: age 35:

1. "I define stress as not being able to find a solution or have an answer. As anger. or people accusing me of something. I feel defenseless. Upset. I feel I need to be able to control my emotions."

2. "Physically, I can't breathe. I have a twisting gut feeling. I get rigid. I walk with my fists clenched. I get depressed more than angry. I think to myself, I messed up. I should be able to control my life, work it out."

Kate: age 30:

1. "Unable to make a good decision."
2. "A big lump in my back, shoulder blades."

Sherry: age 32:

1. "Inability to cope, handle a situation."
2. "Knots in stomach. Can't sleep. Jumpy. On edge."

Belinda: age 39:

1. "I have to pretend everything is o.k. when it's not. I have to hold emotions inside and have a lot things pulling at me and can't get them out into the open."

2. "My tract goes into fits."

Denise: age 39:

1. "Overwhelming sense of inability to complete everything that is required."

2. "Tightness in chest. Tenseness in body, headaches. tightness in shoulders. Stiff neck. Heart palpitations which doctor related to stress."

Debbie: age 38:

1. "All the uncontrollable things in your life."

2. "Headaches. Anxiety. Tight chest. Shortness of breath. Rapid heartbeat. Stomach ache. Loose bowels."

Julie: age 35.

"He personifies stress for me—the minute he walks in the door."

Not every one of these women will develop heart disease, but it is clear their bodies are paying a price for their stress.

Women complaining of chest pain are often told by their physicians to "live with it," or that "it's in your head." Once again, it's the myth at work: doctors have not been trained to think "heart disease" when the patient is female. Part of the problem is that women are more likely than men to experience chest pains not related to heart disease, making their claims easier— if not always justifiably so—to dismiss as something else. That "something else"? A 1987 study at New York's Albert Einstein College of Medicine, asking doctors to diagnose patients with chest pain, found them three times more likely to list the cause as "psychiatric" when the patient was a woman.

The results are often disastrous. As many as one-third of heart attacks in women are never diagnosed. The degree to which untreated angina harms women's hearts is still under study. Well-meaning physicians lament that heart disease in women is simply more difficult to detect. Since women's symptoms often differ from men's, they do not appear to fit the "classic" or "textbook" description and are frequently overlooked. Needless to say, the textbook was developed by studying men; the "book" on women, meanwhile, remains to be written.

Diagnosis, too, is based on the male experience. The stress test, typically one of the first tests given to determine heart disease, has limited usefulness for women. Given that they tend to be older and suffering from other conditions when their symptoms first make themselves known, many women cannot perform the standard treadmill or stationary bicycle exercises necessary for the stress EKG, in which electrodes measure the heart's electrical activity at near-maximum capacity. It almost doesn't matter: two-thirds of the women who do take the test show false positives—indications of coronary disease where there is none. The thallium scan, another first-line diagnostic procedure in which a radioactive isotope, visible on x-ray, is injected into a vein to check blood flow to the heart after exercise, is also flawed—radiologists discovered that women's breast tissue muddies the image.

For these and other reasons, women may never make it to the so-called gold standard of heart-disease tests, angiography. (I got this test in the Emergency Room, after my heart attack.) In angiography, also known as cardiac catheterization, a thin tube is threaded into the heart through a vein or artery, dye is pumped in, and x-rays are taken to look for blocked passages. This is the most accurate of all the tests—but physicians are twice as likely to order it for men with suspected heart disease than for women. One factor in their hesitance is that women's smaller veins increase the chance of complications. But that risk is nothing compared to not performing the test and failing to diagnose a woman's heart disease. Just another reason why prevention is the real gold standard.

Treatment follows the same pattern. Studies have found that men are twice as likely as women to receive aggressive, state-of-the-art care. Women entering emergency rooms with chest pain wait twice as long as men before receiving medical attention. After an attack, they are half as likely to receive the clot-dissolving drugs needed to stave off further damage. Until recent studies touted the benefits of "clotbusters" for all heart-attack sufferers, physicians hesitated to administer them to older patients for fear of bleeding complications. Even so, older men were more apt to receive the drugs than older women. In fact, these drugs do lead to more complications in women—because we have been excluded in the past from tests on their effects and appropriate dosages.

Moreover, delay and neglect when it comes to diagnosis have serious implications on the two aggressive—and potentially life-saving—approaches to treating heart disease: angioplasty and bypass surgery. Women who don't progress to angiography are unlikely to be offered either treatment. By the time they are, they're sicker and the surgery is riskier and usually not advised.

In angioplasty, a catheter with a tiny, deflated balloon on its tip is inserted into the clogged arteries, then inflated to reopen them. Recent studies have found that women referred for this procedure were older and sicker than men—and ten times as likely to die in the hospital from the surgery. But even after risk factors including age, hypertension and diabetes were taken into account, a substantial gap remained: women were four-and-a-half times more likely to die. Experts could not fully explain the disparity, but—stop me if this is becoming familiar—since angioplasty is a technique that was tested and honed on men, the balloons and catheters were made for a man's larger-sized arteries, which could have something to do with it. Recent changes in the technology should help.

No such simple adjustment exists for coronary bypass surgery, in which women's smaller arteries make the operation more difficult and less successful. But again, physiology represents only part of the problem. Women referred for bypass surgery are older and have much more advanced disease than men, with more severe angina and congestive heart failure. By the time they get to the operating table, women are much more likely to require emergency rather than elective surgery, which forces their doctors to use speedier but less favorable methods. As a result of all this, women gain less relief, and die more frequently from the procedure, than men.

Interestingly, recent data suggest that men and women fare equally on their second go-around with heart surgery. This suggests that delayed treatment is the culprit it appears to be. But physicians' concern with statistics showing poorer outcomes for women who have surgery leads many to put it off, further perpetuating the cycle.

A February 25, 1991 study published in the New England Journal of Medicine was among the most extensive and widely reported to find sex differences in coronary angiography, angioplasty, and bypass surgery. Using data from 49,623 patients in Massachusetts and 33,159 in Maryland, the researchers confirmed many of the suspicions raised by previous studies — women admitted to the hospital with myocardial infarction, unstable or stable angina, chronic ischemic heart disease, or chest pain were much less likely to undergo angiography, angioplasty, or bypass surgery. Women who had angina before suffering a myocardial infarction were half as likely to have had angiography to investigate their artery blockage than men with equal or less debilitating angina.

In an accompanying editorial, Dr. Bernardine Healy, then-director of the National Institutes of Health, noted that women in the study who had taken the diagnostic test were just as apt as men to have coronary surgery, and that women who had a myocardial infarction were equally likely to undergo angiography and revascularization. She attributed this to the "Yentl syndrome," after author Isaac Bashevis Singer's 19th-century heroine who was forced to pass herself off as a man in order to attend school and study the Talmud.

"These latter two findings demonstrate the Yentl syndrome at work." Healy wrote. "That is, once a woman showed that she was just like a man, by having severe coronary artery disease or a myocardial infarction, then she was treated as a man would be.

"The problem is to convince both the lay and medical sectors that coronary heart disease is also a woman's disease, not a man's disease in disguise."

Blockage of the arteries is a linear process that starts early; women who aren't careful at a young age are likely to start at a disadvantage when the risks of menopause take hold.

10. risk factors and warning signs

Since the 1960's, intensive public health campaigns have implored men to be kind to their hearts. Don't smoke.... Eat right.... Watch your blood pressure.... These efforts have paid off in a steady decline in the rate of heart disease among men. Women, not targeted in this educational war, have gone the other way.

Simultaneously, research into causes of heart disease in men escalated. It was called an "epidemic." We should be calling women's heart disease also an epidemic, to stimulate the same kind of research and education campaign that was waged for men in the 1960's.

While men have followed their hearts, the myth that heart disease is a male province has left too many women oblivious to basic knowledge that could save their lives—factors that increase their risk, steps they can take to lower their odds, and the symptoms that signal the need for help in the event heart disease strikes.

It's not as if we don't care about our overall well-being. Countless magazines focus on women's health issues, a testament to our interest in the subject. But until a recent upswing, heart disease was conspicuously absent from the popular literature on women and their bodies. So it is that most women are familiar with their family history of breast, ovarian, or cervical cancer, while the disease that kills more of us than all cancers combined goes virtually unnoticed.

Many simply don't think of family history as a risk factor for heart disease. They should think again. Many women also figure they have a free ride at least until menopause, since so few of us suffer heart attacks prior to the so-called change of life. Again, they're wrong—blockage of the arteries is a linear process that starts early; women who aren't careful at a young age are likely to start at a disadvantage when the risks of menopause take hold.

At any age, the facts are these: the more risk factors you possess, the greater your chance of developing heart disease. Added up, the three major controllable risks—smoking, high blood pressure, and high blood cholesterol—multiply by eight a woman's chance of developing heart disease. And if that's not convincing enough evidence that women should care for their hearts as closely as men, we finally have comparative studies to tell us. After decades of male-only prevention research, the first wave of intervention studies involving both sexes has actually found women more amenable to risk-factor influence—both positive and negative—than men. In other words, women respond strongly to being treated and strongly (in a negative fashion) to not being treated. Women who avoid risk factors make a more positive difference in their heart health than men do. It helps women more than men to stop smoking. The other side of the coin: A woman who practices bad habits will elevate her risks more than a man.

Certain risks for heart disease are genetic. Women whose mother or father had a heart attack by the age of 60 are at greater danger. Diabetes, both Type I and Type II, more than doubles a woman's odds, especially in the presence of other risk factors.

And diabetes becomes far more lethal when combined with heart disease in women than in men. Then there's our biological clock: when it expires, whether at natural menopause or hysterectomy (regardless of whether the ovaries are removed), our risk of heart disease doubles, then continues to increase with age—more rapidly, it is believed, than for men.

While we can't stop the clock, there's a great deal we can do—or not do. Let's start with the don'ts.

Smoking: The lungs aren't the only organ damaged by tobacco. Smoking deprives the heart of needed oxygen, harms the artery lining, and invites the blood clots that lead to attacks. Young women who smoke forfeit the natural advantage estrogen provides. If they smoke about two packs a day, their risk is ten times that of nonsmokers.

Tobacco is responsible for nearly half of all heart attacks before age 55, according to a Harvard study. Smokers are less likely to survive an attack. About the only thing worse than smoking is doing so while using oral contraceptives: pairing tobacco use with the birth-control pill sends the odds of an attack skyrocketing. Women on both drugs are *40 times* more likely to suffer a heart attack than women on neither. The good news: quit smoking and your risk plummets to that of a nonsmoker within a couple of years. The bad: while anti-smoking campaigns aimed at men have proved effective, women—untargeted for so long—have continued to embrace tobacco in record numbers. There have yet to be any successful anti-smoking campaigns for women.

Hypertension: High blood pressure—anything above 140/90—is the second of the big-three changeable risk factors, substantially increasing the likelihood of both heart disease and stroke, even at slightly high levels. Hypertension affects more than half of all women in the United states over the age of 55, and two of every three after 65, when a woman's heart-disease danger is already greatest. Most people with hypertension won't know it unless they have their blood pressure measured—it doesn't typically produce symptoms. Among the prescriptions for controlling hypertension: regular exercise, weight loss, and avoidance of alcohol, table salt and sodium. If the problem persists, medication becomes necessary.

High Blood Cholesterol: Approximately one-third of American women have blood cholesterol levels that put them at serious heart-disease risk. A level above 240 is considered "serious," with 200–239 thought to be "borderline—but still enough to boost the odds. The higher the total cholesterol in the blood, the higher the risk: Every one-percent rise portends a two-percent increase in heart-disease prevalence.

Unfortunately, blood cholesterol levels go up with age, especially in women. While young women tend to have lower blood cholesterol than young men, women's average levels climb steadily until their mid-30's then begin a steep trajectory, catching men at about age 45 and then soaring ahead form 45 to 55. By 55, the average total cholesterol level of American women is a precarious 250.

Blood cholesterol is measured in terms of high-density lipoproteins (HDL) and low-density lipoproteins (LDL). HDL, also called "good" cholesterol, helps to keep the lipoproteins from piling up in the blood and narrowing the arteries that transport blood to the heart; LDL does the opposite, mounting as fat. Thus, total blood cholesterol levels don't tell the entire story—what's important, too, is the HDL/LDL ratio. For women, in fact, bad cholesterol may be less of a risk factor than for men, since estrogen is a protector against LDL buildup. But studies have found low HDL ("good" cholesterol) levels to be more dangerous in women than in men—indeed, HDL below 40 is second to age as a predictor that a woman will have heart disease. The best way to reduce overall cholesterol is to cut back on high-fat, high-cholesterol foods. (Cholesterol is found mostly in meat and dairy products.) Weight loss, if you're overweight, also helps, as does quitting smoking and getting exercise. Activity is also thought to be related to higher HDL. (If these methods don't do the trick, physicians may also prescribe cholesterol-lowering medication.)

Obesity: Obesity on its own is a risk factor for women—the more overweight and the older the obese woman, the higher the risk. This would be true independent of the presence of other factors. Of course, obesity (defined as being more than 30-percent above recommended body weight) almost never exists without bringing on other risks. Overweight women, younger than 50, triple their chances of developing hypertension. Obesity also contributes to high blood cholesterol levels and the adult onset of diabetes.

Inactivity: In 1992, the American Heart Association turned the "Big Three" into the "Big Four," placing lack of physical activity alongside smoking, hypertension, and high blood cholesterol. In the largest study on the effects of exercise on female hearts, the most inactive women were found to be at nine times greater risk of dying from heart disease than the most fit. Moreover, even moderate exercise—defined in the study as a brisk daily walk of at least a half-hour—paid handsome dividends.

Which of these got *me?* I didn't smoke. My blood pressure and blood cholesterol levels kept me out of the high-risk category. I exercised moderately and was not obese. I had no family history of heart disease.

The fact is that traditional risk factors fail to explain approximately half of all heart-disease cases. That's why more and more experts are looking at the role of stress.

Talking about reducing stress and actually doing it are two different propositions; sadly, it too often takes a life-changing experience such as mine to take the steps that might have prevented the occurrence in the first place. Perhaps people fail to pull the reins on their stress levels because they don't think it's practical. "Most people can't just 'check out,'" says Dr. Bairey Merz, leaving their work and familial obligations behind. But even without such a major overhaul, a minimal stress-reducing investment can make a monumental difference.

There are two ways to go about it, Dr. Bairey Merz explains. The first is to rid yourself of those particularly stressful aspects of your life that you can. But certain environmental stresses are inevitable. So the second—and perhaps most practical—key to reducing stress is to modify your response to it. She recommends relaxation techniques. "It appears that as little as 15 minutes a day can make an impact," she says. By anyone's definition, minutes well spent.

When simply defined as stimuli, Dr. Bairey Merz notes, stress is something we all have and need—without it, we'd never get out of bed. It becomes a negative based on our reaction to it. "Bad" stress is typically something we create in our own minds; it's how we interpret the world around us. "Unstressed" people tend to be optimistic and flexible, with a strong social-support network of family and friends, a sense that they are basically in control of their lives, and an acceptance of events over which they have no control.

Avoiding the above risk factors substantially improves a woman's outlook, but what about additional steps? Several recent developments are intriguing:

Aspirin: By making it harder for the blood to clot, aspirin appears to have a positive preventive effect. Trouble is, the major studies on the drug's cardiovascular impact have been on men.

Recent research at Harvard Medical School indicates that women, too, are helped by taking one to six aspirin a week, but more studies are needed.

Iron: A large study in Finland—once again done exclusively on 2,000 men—found a strong correlation between high body levels of iron and heart attacks. The results raised several questions for future study: Do low iron levels reduce the risk of attacks? If so, could the practice of bloodletting—draining excess iron from the blood—prove beneficial? And without studying women, they have the temerity to suggest that given that pre-menopausal women lose iron when they menstruate, could this, rather than estrogen, explain their low risk for heart attacks? While far too little is known to come to any of these conclusions, it's worth watching.

Vitamins: Of greater interest is the mounting evidence suggesting a role for certain vitamins in preventing heart disease. The thinking is this: Low-density lipoproteins, the "bad" cholesterol, do their damage through interaction with oxygen. When LDL is oxidized, it lures in other cells and becomes trapped in the arterial walls as plaque. This heart-disease precipitator might never happen, the recent research suggests, if anti-oxidants intervened to nip the plaque-forming process in the bud. In a recent study, women who consumed large amounts of two such anti-oxidants, beta carotene and vitamin E, had lower rates of heart disease than women who consumed smaller amounts.

Estrogen Replacement: More good news comes from studies indicating that post-menopausal women who take estrogen pills dramatically reduce their heart-disease risk, by as much as 50-percent, according to the large Nurses' Health Study at Boston's Brigham and Women's Hospital. The benefit of the pills appears to lie in raising women's HDL levels. Does replacing the hormone lost during menopause enable women to regain their pre-menopausal advantage? Though the evidence is still considered preliminary, other studies have produced similar results.

Several questions remain to be answered. The therapy isn't expected to be right for everyone—studies have found that estrogen replacement increases the risk of breast and uterine cancer. Though the reduction in heart disease risk is likely to far outweigh the therapy's negative effects, women with a family history of breast cancer, for instance, might be advised to steer clear. Another question is whether taking estrogen with the hormone progestin, to counter the uterine-cancer risk, simultaneously blunts the estrogen's benefits to the heart. Further research will also determine when women who are recommended for the therapy should begin, and how long they should stay on it.

Are women more accepting of pain than men? For most of us, personal experience says yes, though it would be difficult to prove. Whether related to biology or sociology, in connection with heart disease this "courage" is not something to brag about.

In a study at the West Virginia University School of Medicine, women averaged four hours from onset of heart-attack symptoms to a call to the hospital; men waited one hour. Because 60-percent of heart-attack deaths occur within the first hour, you can see that women's temperaments are getting them in peril. And, though we are more likely than men to experience angina as a warning sign that heart disease is on the way, we are far less apt to report it—or to recognize the symptoms when they occur.

It makes sense. So little public education on heart-disease symptoms has been aimed at women that it's not surprising when we experience discomfort without suspecting its cause.

And women have been told so many times that their heads are the source of their heart problems it's no wonder when they believe it—and figure they can will their pain away.

Angina typically feels like pressure or squeezing that stretches across the middle of the chest—or like something, in my case an elephant, standing on your chest. The pain or discomfort usually begins after strain, either emotional or physical. It builds gradually, then fades after a few minutes (anything less than a minute is probably not angina; anything longer than a few minutes might signal a heart attack). It can move to other parts of the body, such as the left arm, the jaw, the neck, or the back. Shortness of breath, sweating, nausea and dizziness often accompany the pain.

Don't be a martyr—if you feel as if you might be having a heart attack, call a doctor or go to an emergency room. Men do this all the time. Learn the warning signs. Learn the risk factors. Listen to your heart.

Part Three

But these longings never came to the surface, I was too busy doing what was expected of me.

II. marriage, motherhood and family

After college I withdrew from the early, heady public phase of my life and moved to California to take my chances as a small fish in a big pond. I hadn't wanted to move to California, but that was where my parents moved the family. When I think about it today, the idea of a 21-year-old acquiescing so meekly to her parents astounds me. But I was a product of my time—that's what young women were expected to do. I had been raised not to talk back, and I didn't. Sometimes I still wonder how much anger I swallowed when I remained silent. I boldly made appointments for interviews with managing editors of all five Los Angeles metropolitan daily newspapers— and then dropped down to the suburban dailies. The day of my interview with the Pasadena Star News, I met Joe on a blind date. I had not yet been offered a job, and I was suffering from a damaged ego. I desperately wanted a career, and so I was feeling frustrated.

I don't suppose I had ever felt more self-confident or important than I did when I graduated from the University of Texas. I was twenty-one and I thought I knew everything. Perhaps this is typical of that age. But those unsuccessful job interviews took a lot of starch out of my spine. I felt alone, fearful, and far away from home.

Joe and I had an electric attraction to each other, we viewed the world the same way, we found it easy to talk. I was falling in love and happy to have his help in my job search. Only four weeks after we met we were engaged and six weeks later we were married.

Home to me was Texas—either Mercedes, where I was born and knew I'd never return, or Austin, which I loved and knew I wouldn't stay in either. I wanted to go to New York, to be on top of the pile in journalism. It was a heady time for a young woman to aspire to a newspaper career. Men had gone off to war, leaving behind job openings as writers, reporters, and editors, opportunities heretofore unavailable to women. At that time women distinguished themselves overseas and on the home front as photographers, editors, columnists and reporters.

That's what I wanted. No apprenticeship, no starting at the bottom. Just tell them I had been associate editor of The Daily Texan, show them my clippings, trade on the contacts I had or could muster in New York, and the reputation of our Journalism School, and I'd have no trouble.

One small fact seemed to escape me: those men whose departure created a climate of opportunity for women were returning to reclaim their jobs in the editorial rooms of the nation's newspapers and magazines. There would be no career for me in journalism, especially not starting at the top. I hadn't thought much about radio; and television was still an idea, not a reality.

In many ways the double standard of the work world is duplicated in medical practice and research. Just as the textbook case for heart disease is for men, my early experience in the job market was an experience in which I was always compared to the generic male and never seen as myself. These inequities across the board only add to the stress women experience—the one thing we're supposed to handle like a lady. The pattern of stress remains the same for a woman. Hold it in, function for others. While we do this, minute by minute, imperceptibly, plaque attaches itself to the arteries.

As the excitement of arranging a wedding increased, ideas about work were put on the back burner. I had been offered a job in Pasadena; the only place Joe and I could find to live was in Santa Monica, an hour's drive away in one direction, with his law school almost as far away in another direction. We had only one car. The more we talked about it, the clearer it became that Joe did not want me to work. I called the city editor at Pasadena, whose flunky I was going to be (the textbook version of a flunky is female), and told him I was going to get married, and wouldn't be able to start the job.

I was following my old reaction pattern. I could have arranged to drive to Pasadena if it had been important enough to me. Joe could have taken the street car to USC, although he made a fuss about the few times he had to do it. I could have tried for a job in Santa Monica, in Beverly Hills, in Hollywood. I never thought of it. He didn't want me to work. And so I didn't. I put my needs and my feelings on the shelf.

To compensate, I threw myself into volunteering. In editing my college sorority magazine for a year, I was back to writing, editing, working with the printer to get out a publication. I also joined Hadassah, and edited its newsletter. Part of my work was in solitude, part of it gave me a social toe-hold in my new city.

And there was solitude in my life with Joe, too. He was in his second year of law school and had established a schedule for himself. He went to school five days a week, studied at home every night, and on Fridays, summarized his week's classes with two friends. They had dinner at a restaurant near the campus and worked through the evening. His schedule took precedence, and I was left to fill my time as best I could. He wasn't cruel, but focused on his studies and thus indifferent to my needs; he had what he considered his more serious business to attend to, and I could fend for myself. It was a type of independence, but I had no friends, no confidants, and no husband I could talk to except over dinner. There was, then, nothing to do that I valued. The volunteering was a substitute for a real job; and all the years I volunteered, up to and including high level work in politics. I never felt any ease and recovery from the frustration of not having a meaningful, successful and visible job.

In brief, I wanted my own byline, and I didn't have it.

Early in our marriage, Joe began to talk about having a child. I had no interest in starting a family while he was still in law school, and I still harbored hopes for a career. Still I knew I could count on him. I had no idea what his future would be, but I knew he would take care of me.

What eventually happened was what I considered the worst case scenario. From the first time I met him, Joe's father talked about their practicing law together, and Joe never disputed this course. I hated his father, and I hated the effect he had on Joe and as a consequence, on us as a couple. I hated the idea of his taking for granted that father and son would practice together.

Joe had left home a twenty-one year old kid and returned from the army three-and-a-half years later a mature man with shrapnel in his back and foot, a purple heart and a bronze star. Yet when he practiced law with his father he was treated like a kid. His father was selfish, demanding of attention, uncomplimentary. When he took Joe to court he introduced him as his "sonny boy." It was a partnership in name only; in fact, Joe was an inadequately compensated employee, and this imposed a financial strain on us. Joe had depended on his father to teach him about the practice of law and how to develop a clientele. His father was neither a good law partner nor a good teacher.

I was angry and frustrated that Joe wouldn't separate from his father, stand up for himself, for us. It took three years of their legal partnership and our arguments before I got my point across and Joe went out on his own. This eased a source of friction between us and thus lessened the stress I'd been feeling. By that time we had our first baby. Fourteen months later, we had another. We were poor, but we were independent. Joe paid a big price for this declaration of independence. For the remaining forty-three years of his life his father never forgave him.

This lack of forgiveness was never expressed, only implied. I paid a price for it, too. If they could have ever confronted their unresolved conflicts—either personally or in therapy—they might have been easier together. Almost every day Joe would report some disagreeable, stressful, sometimes painful conversation with his father. (His father called him every day.) Many times I begged Joe to go into therapy. Over the years he had a few sessions; some of them helpful for a time, but he wouldn't hang in long enough to work it out and bring him peace. As many wives do, I became the sounding board for Joe's tension and anger with his dad. And as many wives do, I tried to play a healing role. Most of the time, I'd come out a loser in these talks. I was taking on his stress, making it my own. I was furious that so much of his energy and attention was directed to his relationship with his father, energy and attention I wanted for myself and the children. This surely was one of the building blocks of my stressed female personality.

I threw myself into mothering with great vigor, with a set of goals I tried to realize. I wanted to correct every mistake I thought had been made with me: I wanted to be a present mother, rather than an absent, working mother, as I perceived mine had been. I wanted to give my children freedom, not put many strictures on their development. I wanted them to learn to express their feelings. It was called "being permissive" in those days. And yet, I never could quite figure out how to balance letting the boys have freedom to learn, to experiment and to grow, and at the same time to give them some boundaries and some discipline. Many times I remember screaming out in frustration.

As Joe remembers it, he was an active parent. I don't remember it that way. He took up tennis, and after his Saturday morning game he would eat lunch and lie down to rest; I would keep the children quiet so they wouldn't disturb Daddy. Until he woke up, I would also entertain his parents, who came to visit us every Saturday, putting aside the hurt between father and son. I would walk on eggs to avoid conflict, to keep spirits high. Of course, I wasn't relaxed. It never occurred to me to think, let alone say, "I want to take every Saturday afternoon off." I might have enjoyed shopping—though I couldn't have afforded to buy anything—or visiting a friend or my family or going to the beach by myself. But these longings never even came to the surface. I was too busy doing what was expected of me.

More than forty years later, lumps form in my throat when I think back to those painful times. I began to have stomach aches, and Bill Molle, our doctor, advised me to go out and do something for myself. By then I had a cleaning lady, and when she came I went out; but only once do I remember an uncharacteristic outing for myself—a swim at the Ambassador Hotel pool. It never crossed my mind that Joe should take a part in child rearing or give me relief. He worked hard all week; he needed a rest.

Nevertheless, I learned to be a good mother. I felt creative and rewarded. I was working, but I didn't have a regular job. and I didn't have any bylines, either.

Then two family stories—two traumas—became my trauma, my stress—for life.

A Daughter's Stress

My father had moved to California in 1946 to set up a business with my cousins. Although he totally financed the enterprise, he made them equal partners; however, within a few years, my cousins relegated this once successful businessman to a flunky's position and began a campaign to take the business away from him.

He fought back. It was a great embarrassment to my father to engage in a legal dispute with family, but finally, the business was dissolved, and my parents moved to Los Angeles. A short period of relative calm set in—but soon anxiety crept in. The lack of activity overwhelmed this man unprepared for retirement. In desperation, he purchased a shoe store in a failing section of downtown Culver City, while all over America businesses were moving away from central Main Streets to new malls. His thinking was frenetic at that time. We didn't know how frenetic until later. He overstocked the store, trying to put a good face on a bad decision. I remember going there one day with Fred, a thirteen-month-old toddler, and seeing shoe boxes stacked to the ceiling in a small narrow shop, shoe boxes crowded into the aisles in the rear of the store. I felt that everything would crash down on my head, an eerie premonition of danger.

I was pregnant with David. A few weeks later he was born; I had two babies, a new house, a husband unhappy in law practice with his father, and my father showing signs of an instability we didn't understand.

By late March, Daddy collapsed with a deep depression, unable to move. A psychiatrist administered shock treatments, something used in 1951 just before anti-depressant drugs were introduced. Mother told us how Daddy's body contracted and convulsed and then seemed to release and relax after the treatments. I don't know how many treatments he had. Maybe not enough. He didn't get well.

A psychiatrist came to my father's bedside and asked him if there was anything wrong with his marriage. Neither his Germanic personality nor his line of inquiry were acceptable to my father. That anyone should question the quality of their relationship was an insult neither of my parents would tolerate. Daddy threw him out of the house.

So there he lay, without treatment. My mother, a strong and determined woman who, until the day she died, believed in the power of positive thinking, thought she could help my father back to health by loving him, by talking to him, by taking care of him. She rejected the idea that anyone else could help him. We were warned that Daddy's severe reaction depression made suicide entirely possible. The doctor told us to keep knives, razors, medications away from him. I don't know if he suggested institutionalization, I think not; and I suspect that mother in her strength, bordering on arrogance, would have refused.

One rainy April morning, Daddy persuaded Mother to go to the shoe store to see how business was going. She left him alone for about an hour. That was all it took. When she returned home and couldn't find him, she called me in desperation to see if I knew where he was, and left me waiting on the phone while she went out to look for him. Joe raced back over the short distance to their home. They found him. Hanging from the rafter in the garage, with the rope from the clothesline wrapped around his neck in a perfect noose. For some bizarre reason, I stayed on the phone, calling, "Mother, Mother," but she didn't answer.

Even with the warnings, my father's suicide was something we had never contemplated. He was only fifty-one, mother was forty-seven, we were a young family—I was twenty-six, my sister twenty-four, my brothers twenty and seventeen. We were as bewildered as we were bereaved. I felt this as a literal weight on my heart.

In my search for enlightenment I learned that electroconvulsive therapy, shock treatment, introduced in 1938 and nearly abandoned in the 1960's was 95 percent effective and constituted the first treatment method which could reliably end episodes of major depression.

In those first years after Daddy died, I read everything I could about mental illness. After I went into therapy, mostly to deal with the sibling rivalry problem, I began to understand more about the nature of depression and suicide. As I have matured, there have been many times that I wondered if depression was an inheritable trait, whether in my depressed periods, I could have been capable of such an aberration. Wondering about it made me determined to face head-on whatever problems I had, not to resort to a solution that would injure my family for the rest of their lives.

The stress from his death gurgled underneath the surface of my life for years. My father's death left me with a void, a vast empty space in my understanding of him and our relationship.

I postponed telling my children. Finally when they were young teenagers, it was a relief to tell them and to escape from the stigma I had associated with his death.

And what effect did it have on me? First, it made me keenly aware of mental illness and sensitive to the signs of it in anyone I knew, including myself. It made me sympathetic to psychological treatment, comfortable using it to help myself and willing, if not anxious, to recommend it for members of my family.

A Mother's Stress

When I was thirty-three a life-changing event took place: unexpectedly I became pregnant with our third child. What had started as a year of high hopes, a sense that the boys were well-launched, happy, old enough and sufficiently independent for me to consider exploring new paths and pursuing my own interests, ended with a pregnancy filled with lethargy and preoccupation with my own health. After I attended to the needs of my family, I spent hours in bed; I took questions about health to my obstetrician, who told me I was psychologically rejecting this baby, and to drink orange juice when I felt faint in the grocery store. He did not tell me to eliminate salty foods or reduce whatever it was that was causing my toxemia; he was hung up on psychiatry and thought my symptoms were psychosomatic.

Sarah's delivery was uncomplicated, the doctor put a tiny, three-pound, thirteen-ounce, sixteen-inch-long baby girl on my abdomen, and said, "I'm glad she's out of there." She was full term, strong enough to breathe on her own, but was placed in an isolette for warmth. On the birth certificate, under complications, the doctor wrote, "Toxemia in a mild form." I thought it vindicated the months of feeling wretched, never being put on a special diet, never an acknowledgment that there might have been a physical basis for my complaints.

Sometime in the middle of the night, within an hour of delivery, I had a convulsion, unattended. The next day, when Joe and my mother were visiting me, the room began to spin before my eyes and I shook into a second convulsion.

Luckily, the senior resident in the department, Dr. Walter Fox, who had interned at Los Angeles County Hospital and had seen many cases of toxemia and postpartum eclampsia (the convulsions), rushed into the case and saved my life. I had already bitten a deep gash into my tongue and injured my shoulder on the bed rail the night before.

The poisons I had complained about, building and circulating in my body during pregnancy, had caught up with me, knocked me out, separated me from my baby, from myself, from my husband and mother, and from my two little boys at home, waiting, longing for their mother, not understanding what was happening to her across town. I'm not sure to this day what Joe told them, but nobody had an explanation for it at that time.

After the second convulsion, I lapsed into a coma, unable to nurse Sarah, to hug her, to care for her, or bond to her in any way. When I came back to life, I asked for my baby; I needed to know her. What had she experienced? I knew that I couldn't nurse her as I had planned, I could not give her sustenance. I remembered nothing. Unseen doctors and nurses, the strength in my soul, my will to live and God's grace saved me.

I believed the toxemia that almost took me away from Sarah at birth, and almost took her away from me, caused her dangerously low birth weight. I wouldn't learn the truth until Sarah was over thirty.

When Sarah was one-and-one-half, the pediatrician noticed a heart murmur. He listened for a year before he told me about it, and said it was time to have a cardiogram as a first step in diagnosing the condition. I was in a daze, but tried to act nonchalant to give her courage, to keep from her the anxiety I felt.

Here was my reaction to stress, working full time. I made a stupid personal decision: to handle this information myself, not to tell Joe, because he was suffering from a bad back, a candidate for surgery, and didn't need any more pressure. I would handle it myself. Many months later, after I told him, we promised each other we wouldn't play that game again, but over the years, both of us have played it repeatedly to protect the other. We are better at being honest with each other now than we were in those days.

Sarah's first heart catheterization at Children's Hospital confirmed the diagnosis of congenital aortic stenosis, a narrowing of the aortic valve.

I never slept soundly again. Every night I would awaken, creep into her room to listen for her breathing. And I knew that every day of my life after that I would worry about Sarah dying, dying of heart disease.

Given easily to respiratory infections, Sarah suffered numerous bouts of croup, and during one especially bad session, we took her to Children's Hospital again to be placed into a tiny crib encased in a plastic tent where cool vapor mist circulated to help relieve the wheezing, coughing and choking. I spent the nights with her at the hospital, leaning into the misty environment to comfort her, to persuade her to stay inside the tent. She looked up beseechingly to me. I couldn't heal her, but I could help her tolerate the treatment that would. I didn't realize it at the time, but this would be a theme that would unite us on her life's path.

Within another year, Sarah was back in the hospital for an operation to correct a strabismus that caused her eye to drift off center to the left. Nothing serious, easily attended to in the hands of experts. Again, I spent my nights with her in the hospital. Before Sarah was five, she had been a hospital patient three times. I developed a studied nonchalance and casual acceptance of circumstances and conditions as they presented themselves. I didn't want to keep myself at the edge of hysteria and I didn't want Sarah to become a hypochondriac, but to accept these developments as easily as her small frame and blue eyes. I tried to pass this acceptance along to Sarah, and in some ways I think I succeeded. I was bottling up my own stress.

She was an extremely articulate child, she crawled and walked within normal age range. But Sarah was sending out conflicting developmental signals: she knocked over cups of milk regularly, she had red scraped knees and bruised shins from stumbling, she developed a shyness, and always withdrew from the group to play in the doll and housekeeping corner of her nursery school. She had a very short attention span, didn't use paint brushes well or learn to cut with scissors, never learned to swing herself, and avoided tricycles and wheel toys. I began to see that her coordination and physical development were coming along too slowly. I had never seen a child quite like her and I began a search for answers. The pediatrician was very little help. I was on my own to read, to research, to learn, and to experiment.

We enrolled Sarah in a day camp organized to serve children of differing developmental needs, and for the first time Sarah was in the company of handicapped and dysfunctional children. Fred and David, who accompanied me to pick her up at camp, were horrified to see her in such a group. I saw her withdrawing into herself as she became aware of the differences between herself and her handicapped playmates in camp as well as the "normal" kids in the nursery school and in the neighborhood. At the end of Sarah's first school year, they wanted her to repeat kindergarten, she was holding her books upside down, and wasn't able to keep up with the other children.

Joe and I asked for a conference with the principal and the supervisor of the western district of the Los Angeles school system. They said they had never seen a child like this. But they had no suggestions.

We could not believe our ears, never seen another child like that?—with their experience? We were horrified, rudderless, without resources or clues of where to turn for help. As planned, we moved to a new house in another school district, but not before I consulted with the new principal. She promised to watch over Sarah, and when they saw her drifting behind, she said, "If Sarah were my child, I'd have her tested from the tips of her toes to the top of her head to diagnose her problem."

After a battery of tests and numerous consultations, we enrolled Sarah in a small, specialized private school, the Frostig School, where she could also receive psychological counseling as she experienced some success in learning and development. Sarah had learning difficulties, including dyslexia, and small and large muscle motor coordination problems—both interrelated in their view—which would be dealt with together in the school. Finally, we felt we had found a protective, nourishing learning environment for Sarah.

We were pioneers, she was a pioneer. So as all pioneers do, we struck out onto uncharted paths. In those days, neither lay people nor professionals spoke of dyslexia, learning disabilities or special education; the truth is, little was known.

What had begun as a probable one-and-a-half years, stretched all through the elementary school grades, accompanied by psychological therapy. Sarah's education was on several levels, academic, physical, and ability training. She worked in a highly specialized atmosphere. Although the umbilical cord had been cut at Cedars of Lebanon in 1958, it seemed to have remained intact during the early school years, stretched long for the purpose of moving out of my range, but a tether, nonetheless. She was dependent on me. And I was overprotective. I made her education and growth my new career, reading everything I could about learning disabilities, showing so much understanding, concern and involvement that I almost shut Joe out of the process.

I had this push and pull relationship with Sarah, wanting to support her, wanting to encourage her and, at the same time, wanting to push her out of the nest. Over the years, I never knew if Sarah's progress and behavior was because she couldn't or because she wouldn't. There were moments when I respected her rhythm; but many more times I remember screaming at her in frustration about her dependence, her unwillingness to confront difficult social situations. Sarah would never walk through any open door for the first time unless she was holding firmly to my hand. It was a question of whether I wanted her to have the experience on the other side of the door—either with failure or success—or to stand and wait and see if she would go through alone. I chose to accompany her, through her childhood and teen years. I wasn't doing her, or myself, any good in those outbursts.

Joe had a stubborn faith in Sarah, believed that she was smarter than she was testing, always reasoning she could do better. He was at once supportive and frustrated. But he must have conveyed his faith in her, although he found it very hard to cope with her behavior of dependence, clinging and physical fragility. I wasn't in therapy at the time, but I was reading a lot, and I was going through one of my half-cocked Freudian phases where I thought it would be detrimental to Sarah if she sat on her father's lap beyond a certain age or had too close a physical contact. The most natural thing for Joe was to embrace, to hug, to kiss, to touch; it was what Sarah needed most of all, and I, in my highmindedness, discouraged it. Needless to say, it was a time of intense conflict and tension in our family. It was as if so much energy was concentrated on Sarah that the boys had to grow up alone. But I couldn't allow that; I was a fiercely committed mother, a highly energetic, project-driven woman determined to do the best I could with and for my kids. It meant a lot of juggling. And a lot of stress. Stress, too, from the 1960's and 1970's—the years of drug experimentation, the Vietnam war, and young people's rejection of their parents' values.

Through her strength and determination, Sarah finished junior and senior high school and two years of college. With our insistence and her acquiescence, she was willing to go away from home, to live with a number of roommates, all of them unsatisfactory, who have taken advantage of her and sometimes abused her, but her resilience and strong survival instincts sustained her. It's as if the strength she showed us upon delivery, where this tiny baby had the strength to breathe on her own and needed only warmth to survive, had been a hallmark of her persona. But her independence has not been easily achieved; it has been won with slow, painstaking steps, sometimes, seemingly, more losses than gains.

The early years were years of intense stress for all of us, and years of growth, insight and understanding we never could have known without her.

Now Sarah lives alone, manages her own life, works as an assistant teacher in a pre-school and has earned her certificate in early childhood education. A success story of love and perseverance and great self-respect and courage on her part.

In January 1994, Sarah was knocked out of bed by the earthquake. We moved her home with us to escape the severely damaged, uninhabitable condo.

In March 1994, on an annual cardiac examination, Sarah was told that she had developed symptoms in her aortic stenosis that required immediate open heart surgery. Fortunately, when the surgeon went in, he found something that couldn't be seen on any monitoring measure, it could only be seen in surgery, that her aortic narrowing was just below the valve, sub-aortic stenosis. He cut out the encroaching membranes and did not have to replace the valve. This meant that she would not be on blood thinning medication the rest of her life and that she could have children. Sarah made a remarkable, uneventful recovery. She has more energy now than she has ever had. And she has no fears about her heart.

Finally, neither do we.

Women should find their feelings first and then their mouths to express them.

12. travels with Joe

I think the major part of my stress in the ten years before my heart attack came from dealing with Joe's explosion onto the public scene as the star/judge of his television show, "The People's Court." There was a sense of unreality when Joe auditioned for the role and shot the pilot. I had insisted from the beginning (here I was, minding his business) that he be absolutely certain his reputation as a fair and fine judge for twenty years would not be jeopardized by this new venture. I urged him to consult with leading members of the California Bar and Bench, people whose opinions he valued. From what Joe told them of the plans, they gave him a green light to go ahead.

I was still working and struggling with a personal decision: whether to retire or continue work. I had begun to travel with Joe on promotional trips and felt that I could play a role in the travels, to watch over Joe's level of fatigue and excitement, and to act as the traveling public relations consultant. Even with the travel and interrupted schedule, I maintained my work load exactly as before. Juggling was becoming a strain.

The second winter of the show, Joe and I went on a vacation cruise. Across the dinner table, I said, "I'm having a terrible time with this decision and I need your help. What do you think about my retiring?"

"If you do, don't expect me to be your playmate," he said.

Tears ran down my cheeks, because he had so badly missed the point of my question. Instinctively I knew if I quit work, I would be losing my separate identity. But if I didn't quit, I would be imposing almost inhuman stress on myself. Tongue-tied, I couldn't explain this to him that night.

From the beginning, I felt I was playing a role in Joe's celebrity and travel life. I was protecting him, I was also protecting my marriage by my presence at his side, and I was helping him keep the adulation in some perspective. Perhaps I was protecting myself, too. I didn't want the entire focus of our life together to revolve around his fame and the stories that were associated with his show or his popularity; and I didn't want too much "judgieness" at home. I fought hard against using our dinner table as a bench from which he could preside, and I didn't want to surrender to that now. But I was paying a price, and it came upon me so suddenly and forcibly that I couldn't ignore it.

During the years of the show, I had good times, funny times, wonderful close times with Joe. In our private moments, we laughed and marveled at this new happening. But our private moments were few.

Without doubt, the funniest fan was a waitress in Reno. She ran across the room, pencil and pad poised to take the order and suddenly took a running dive and jumped into our booth, almost on Joe's lap.

"You know what I like about you, Judge Wapner? You don't take any shit from any of them," she said.

And I have had some very painful years of personal insult, rarely intentional, just a side effect of being the spouse of a celebrity. In the early years, when I was wanting very much to write, I considered writing a book. "Out of the Spotlight," where I would talk about my feelings and also interview mates of famous people who had also been personages in their own right, but had been standing beside the loved partner, just outside the spotlight. I could even envisage the cover art on the book jacket, a couple holding hands and the spotlight falling around him, her body completely in the shadows. I had gathered names of couples in many fields, sports, entertainment, literature, medicine. But when it came right down to writing it, I could not allow myself to go public.

Even in press, radio and television interviews when I was occasionally asked questions, I learned it was mere tokenism; they did not want to hear an honest answer from me. One day in Baltimore I began a frank response to a TV reporter's question, but he interrupted me mid-sentence and turned the questioning back to Joe.

I have grown in my role, and I have learned to protect myself—sometimes by not going along on interviews—so that when someone asks me how it feels to be married to Judge Wapner, I flash a big smile and say, "Wonderful!" Once I learned to leave the hurt feelings at home and plan ahead for the questions, I could answer questions with humor.

"How is it at home, married to a judge?" I would be asked.

"We don't have any judging at home," I said.

If I am present, and the reporter wants to interview me after finishing with Joe, I will be asked how long we have been married, how many children we have, how it is to live with Joe, and how our lives have changed since "The People's Court." As far as I can ascertain, there is nothing in these questions which might reveal what kind of person I am, what, if anything, I have ever done in my life besides being married to Joe and having children, and the obvious voyeuristic interest in how celebrities live. It is hard for them to handle my responses: that we have had the same friends for forty years, and aside from the traveling and public attention, our personal lives have changed very little. It is a question of values, and that is too philosophical a question to deal with—never possible in quick radio and TV sound bites, not good for the entertainment section of the print media. Besides, as I have had to learn, they are not interested in me, what I was, who I am, what I think. Early on, I fooled myself into thinking that this information might give a more rounded picture to the life of Judge Wapner. I learned it was not to be. The special partnership that we enjoyed, our interdependence, did not interest them.

One day about the fourth year, I told Joe that I had been having an especially hard time with his fame and feeling left out. I had been humiliated by being ignored and by becoming a nonperson. I told him it wasn't any of his doing, but that he had to know what I had been feeling, that I had tried to be a good sport and go along with it, but I was deeply pained and wanted him to know about it. I thought the best thing for me was to drop back and try to stay away from accompanying him to all public appearances, be selective. It was a relief to level with Joe.

I had thought if I complained or did anything less than putting on a good face, I would cramp his enjoyment of this phenomena that had occurred. He said he had tried to include me, introduce me, and I knew that he had. Many times, he would take my hand and draw me to his side, and begin to introduce me, only to have me muscled aside and ignored. It wasn't any of his doing, it was the nature of his becoming a public property, with his viewers feeling they had claims on all his time no matter where and when they encountered him.

It was a matter of how I responded. I took it to heart. Another woman would have loved it. But it was back to that old male-female thing, she supporting him in his upward trajectory. I have heard a country western song "You were the wind beneath my wings," purportedly a love song and tribute to his woman. I would like to have written and recorded a painful lament for the woman to sing in chorus.

We had established a habit of traveling together, and Joe didn't want to go out of town without me; and I began to stay in the hotel while he went out on interviews, and that eased things a bit.

As I thought about my life with Joe as a celebrity, I never wanted to be a co-star. I just wanted to be a person. And I still didn't have my own byline.

During the early years of "The People's Court," I had the feeling that we were gone all the time. There was just enough time to unpack and get things in and out of the cleaners; pack again; get the mail, personal telephone calls, and grooming needs taken care of before we were off again. It seemed to me that we rarely had time to go to the theater, to a concert, to dinner with friends and family.

And during this same period, Mother was failing. Both siblings and Joe and I had become troubled with Mother's disorientation, garbled speech, lurching, stumbling gait, and sudden decline in vision. One night when we were in Washington, D.C., I remember a series of telephone calls back and forth across the country to Leisure World and to UCLA Medical Center where Mother was admitted. We became students of medicine, as doctors explained and diagrammed their evaluations. They concluded that she had an undiagnosed infection of the central nervous system. and thereafter, we always referred to her condition this way.

Knowing the name of it was not going to change anything. It was an important lesson for me to learn: there are medical conditions without explanation or treatment. We had to accept it. Accepting it that day, made it much easier for me to understand and to bear my mother's decline as the years went on.

Joe has always contended that my obsession with Mother's condition caused me the stress that struck to my arteries; neither my psychiatrist nor I think so. As I think about those times, perhaps there is some truth in his contention, but I felt I was handling Mother's illness in a timely and accepting way. No delays were allowed, no ignorance informed our actions, most times I took charge of the medical care and the household help, in consultation with my siblings.

I have examined my childhood, my growing up years, my early marriage and child rearing years, as well as the effect of my mother's illness on my stresses, to try to identify possible plaque development. If my goal, to help other women understand the causes of stress in their lives is to be fulfilled, I need to be perfectly honest with myself and my readers, to also explore my relationship with my husband.

Joe is my best friend, a loving, a most adoring husband, and we have grown and learned together over a long marriage. I am still trying to learn, particularly about my reaction to our almost predictable behavior together. Millions of people know Joe and his behavior on "The People's Court." He is successful because of his skill, his legal, judicial and life experiences, his engaging personality, his sense of humor, his good looks, his fairness and his honesty, and he is willing to reveal his true character daily to millions of strangers. What I have to say about him will not come as a surprise to those who know him. As many of our friends have said, "What you see is what you get" with Joe.

Joe is very smart, quick, a bit bombastic and short tempered. He needs to come rapidly to a conclusion. He sees things in black and white. He has a great need to be in control of himself—so as not to lose his temper—and of people and events around him.

Howard Rosenberg, Pulitzer Prize-winning television critic for the *Los Angeles Times*, recently wrote, ". . . after Judge Joseph Wapner had made a ruling on 'People's Court' concerning a monetary spat that two squabbling girl-friends had earlier tried to resolve during a lunch at Bob's Big Boy.

"He was awesome.

"Fierce. Uncompromising. Tough. Explosive. Irritating. Insulting. Fearless. Intolerant of fools. Sharp-tongued. Tyrannical. Fanatically focused. All-knowing. Absolutely, flat-out terrifying.

"Yes, no one of sound mind would dare cross paths with Wapner."

As much as we have in common, we are two distinct and separate personalities. When he makes a simple, human mistake, he feels grossly incompetent and is angry with himself. He behaves in a grumpy manner. Or if there is something between us, he withdraws in silence to sort it out alone. Only then can we clear the air.

I, on the other hand, need to talk things through. Though I am stubborn, judgmental and impatient when things go wrong, I tend to get over it more quickly.

I have a need to help Joe understand why something that has gone wrong for him is not a huge calamity, but one of the rhythms of life. My "mothering" attempts invariable infuriate him.

These long silences have hung like a pall between us over all the years of growing and learning together, possibly depositing their residue as plaque in my arteries as I bottled up the rage and swallowed the anger. I have blamed his father for his influence in shaping Joe's behavior, although I know Joe has fought hard not to replicate his father's ways.

Over the years, Joe and I have differed in our opinions, sometimes on trivial issues, sometimes on important ones. Earlier, when we disagreed, each of us felt we were right; and if that were the case, the other must be wrong. It was part of our personalities, part of needing to assert control over the other. It always led to anger, hurt; it never ended well. (I always thought I was the loser because I would either give in or be beaten down by Joe's persistence.)

I have since learned that I can avoid conflict if I accept the fact that we both don't have to see things the same way. If we look at things differently, then there's no right or wrong, there's no wining or losing, there's no one in control. We don't need to be alike. I thought so for many years. Now I don't. I can allow for the differences.

If I had been able to look at things that way many years ago, I would have saved myself a lot of grief, spending lonely days and nights not speaking, each locked in the same position. Stress likely would have been reduced in our lives. If I had been able to assert my own place, my own position, my own needs, things would have been a lot easier.

Lately, and particularly since the heart attack, I have learned some techniques for modifying my behavior. I have tried to stop solving Joe's problems, learned to walk away during those bouts of what I consider bad behavior and busy myself with other things until he comes back. Sometimes I have to be willing to stretch this out for a day or two, even a week. I have told him that his behavior was unacceptable, that I wasn't going to put up with it anymore, that I was taking good care of myself, doing what I was told to do, eating carefully, taking my medications, exercising, but the one thing I did not know how to do was to quantify my stress, and I was not going to take any more of it from him.

Some would say I am describing typical male and female behavior in conflict. Maybe so, and there is a large literature on the subject of relations between the sexes, but that is not good enough for me. Women should not put up with disagreeable behavior; they should find their feelings first and then their mouths to express them. It will be healthier for both in the relationship.

I notice lately that Joe is able to meet a conflict or shortcoming with more equanimity and to recover and forgive himself more readily. We are still learning together. And still taking care of each other. And still loving each other. Very deeply.

Some Tips on Reducing Stress in a Relationship:

    Don't mind your husband's business.

    Stop and listen.

    When you think you're juggling too many roles and responsibilities, choose those most important to you. Drop the others.

    Don't take things to heart.

    Remember: you and your husband are distinct and separate personalities.

    Don't try to "mother" your husband.

    You and your husband don't have to see things the same way.

    Stop trying to solve your husband's problems.

    Don't put up with disagreeable behavior.

A balanced, moderate lifestyle—and good coping mechanism—must be good for your heart.

13. I am now older and wiser

When Fred and David were under five, I was having a tough time dealing with their conflicts and constant fighting, and wanted desperately to spare them the sibling rivalry pain I had suffered with my sister. Every week I took books out of the library to read up on the phenomenon, to learn something in the hope of helping them and making life easier on myself. I must not have read enough or the right things to learn how normal sibling rivalry is. (Current child rearing books give parents insight I could have used then and suggestions about easing these conflicts, a help for both parents and children.)

THERAPY

I was really desperate for help and it was at that time I first went into therapy. The stresses of my life up to this time and thereafter may seem irrelevant or minor compared to others whose lives appear, to them, threatened. I am not laying claim to the most stressful of lives; what I am saying is that these are my stresses and I have taken them to heart. I did not develop mechanisms for dealing with these stresses or pressures as they came to me; therefore they were unrelieved. My instinctive response was to take it all in, to take it to heart, to put a good face on things, act agreeable, appear to accept. I did not develop an outward rebellious streak; nor did I ever participate in sports or exercise, either one of which would have relieved stress. I never learned to play.

Perhaps it was a generational response; many women I have spoken with attest to similar behaviors as they were growing up, from childhood and into their adult years. "This is the way we were supposed to behave," many have told me.

I kept pushing on to succeed, never realizing my own expectations nor developing a strategy, technique or philosophy for dealing with failures, frustrations, or people who appeared to get in my way. As I encountered these stumbling blocks, I may have seen myself as victim, rarely as part of the problem. Not an attractive characteristic; also not comfortable to live with.

These reaction patterns were not serving me well. My relationship with my husband and kids was volatile. All I could do was seek professional counseling at different stages of my life. First, I sought help to deal with my sons' sibling rivalry and early strains in my marriage, later for help with Sarah during her school years, for my wild mood swings in early menopause, for guidance in relating to my grown children as adults, and, finally, for post cardiac crisis counseling. Everyone who has gone into therapy knows that treatment is rarely limited to the precipitating cause, so I went back and forth in time, down into and around the formative and influential patterns in my life.

These therapies were for different purposes and with different therapists. I had analytic psychotherapy with two psychiatrists and one PH.D. clinical psychologist, and therapy with two social workers, one very confrontational. Each helped create an atmosphere where I could dig deep into myself to find my pain and articulate my feelings, and sometimes develop strategies and relief and solving problems.

Each of them helped me grow to new plateaus of understanding myself, my relationships with my family, my response to stresses in my life. I learned to value and practice my rights as an individual; I learned appropriate ways to respond to troublesome situations and persons; I learned to speak up. With it all I still had my basic nature, and though I backslid many times, I could recognize my responses and make quicker mid-course corrections.

As I look back, I couldn't have dealt with my problems in any other way. But as I see my life in the context of my heart attack and new knowledge, I know I would subscribe to a broader approach. Therapy, yes, but also augmented by behavior modification strategies, meditation and exercise.

I undertook this retrospective evaluation of my stresses to try to understand what part they played in the development of my heart disease, to share and to encourage others—women in particular—to look objectively at their lives, their stresses, and their responses, so they can keep their juices flowing and their blood pumping and their arteries clean and open. I'm sure there are no guarantees, but a balanced, moderate lifestyle—and good coping mechanisms—must be good for your heart.

But for all of their expertise and all the help I received, I realize today that not one of the therapists that I consulted ever said to me, "Your behavior is not good for your health."

If they had, I like to think that I would have paid attention, and that I might have felt some urgency to change more, perhaps take things less to heart, with less understanding than with traditional methods. Perhaps neither health professionals nor therapists were making those connections until recently.

Aging

The first time I really felt old was when I hurt my back on the fourth of July weekend, 1976—the year of our Bicentennial, the year of the Olympics, and the year Sarah went to

Israel. I carried out to the curb large, heavy loads of newspapers for recycling, and then I made the twin beds for my visiting Israeli cousins. That was the proverbial last straw. Just as I was leaning over to tuck the sheet into the far corner, against the wall, a vicious pain grabbed my back and ran down my leg. I collapsed on the floor. I could not get up. I crawled and pulled myself to my room. I couldn't walk, I couldn't attend to myself. I was put to bed for about two months, until I felt better. I felt as if I might never be able to return to self-sufficiency and independence. I felt awful and I looked awful. I was 51. Until that moment, I had thought that 51 was young.

By the time I got to my mid-fifties, I had a doctor for every orifice: ears, nose and throat; gynecologist; urologist; proctologist. What needed fixing, they fixed. I had had two breast biopsies for the cysts in my breasts; no cancer. I had a hemorrhoidectomy.

I believed in preventative medicine, so there were a lot of doctors in my life. I also had my internist for regular check-ups, occasionally, a dermatologist for assorted spots and bumps, to take the spidery purple blotches out of veinal legs, to inject my sun-damaged nose, and to freeze the growing number of brown sun-damaged spots on my hands and face. As each deterioration appeared, I went good naturedly about its repair, never really associating it with aging. I suppose the energy and vitality of my life counterbalanced those creeping occurrences. I don't know where my head was. Numbers didn't seem to register in my mind. However, as I entered each decade of my life, I was deeply depressed.

Now I have a theory that elderly persons' social lives revolve around visiting their doctors.

My thirties I saw as the end of youth, and I saw it as an end of innocence, too. During my thirties, I devised a game that I have played in all the decades since. I decided I was in my early thirties until I was thirty-four. Not till I got to thirty-five was

I in my mid-thirties. And I stayed in my mid-thirties till about thirty-eight-and-a-half.

It was the same during my forties, fifties and now sixties. The hardest decades to turn the calendar on were the thirties, forties and fifties. When I turned sixty, I felt so marvelous, I thought that I looked the same as earlier, and felt I had achieved a certain level of comfort and ease in my life—even a measure of wisdom and understanding—and I looked forward to the decade. I would examine the lines in my face and decide I would not have a face lift. I was more interested in liposuction to remove the fat from my hips; it was the influence of California, the plastic surgery capital and vanity center of the world. Joe was horrified with either idea. And he was the best possible husband to have. He thought I was beautiful. What more could I want?

In her last years, when her memory was mostly gone, my mother would ask me how old she was, and each year from eighty-three, to eighty-four, eighty-five, eighty-six, and eighty-seven, when I told her, she would sit silently, absorbing the number, tilt her head to the side, repeat the unbelievable age, and say "Hmm, no wonder I can't do what I used to, I'm getting to be a little old lady."

It was dear and sweet of her, and it gave me a chance to talk to her about what a full and healthy life she had lived and how she was declining and needed to accept it. I was hoping to reduce the terror she was feeling at her incompetence, although she couldn't talk about it, but the look in her eyes and the depression in her body and spirit told me that whatever part of her was remembering and functioning, she didn't like what was happening to her.

Life and death hold us by the hand as we go through life, one pulling forward, one pulling back, each pulling in opposite directions. Death will always win in the end, of course, but it occasionally tugs even as life holds on.

Ah, the trick is to learn how one pulls against the other. To encourage one, hold the other at bay, if we can, and sometimes ignore death's signals, squeezing life's-held hand tighter. Perhaps it is this trying to hold death at bay, squeezing life's hand harder that is the feeling of aging that I am now so keenly feeling.

If I looked younger and felt younger, wouldn't that mean death was farther away? I lay in bed with death and hardly knew it was there. When I awakened to life, I wanted by, whatever means, to push death out of that bed. And I have. But as I look at my aging face and sagging body and know that no young man would love it, and that the man who loves it is also old, then I know I am losing the strength to hold life's hand tighter than death's. And as I need to rest and show the definite lessening of energy, I know my youthfulness is still at home only in my mind. After the heart attack, I felt depleted, afraid, incapable of strength of body or spirit, but I didn't think of it as aging, I only thought of it as a God-given postponement of death, a new life.

I seem to have become preoccupied with aging, almost to the point of depression. I desperately wanted to come to acceptance, to transcendence, to live my life with equanimity. Little by little I have. I know that I will not travel to all the places that were on my list. First of all, I am still afraid to go where medical services are not top notch and instantly available. Secondly, I know I don't have the energy to tramp around from morning till night without pause. But I am not going to give up travel altogether; I will modify my list and my pace.

I'm not going to hear all the music, but I have heard more concerts and seen more operas than in all my life before the heart attack. I'm not going to read everything I want, and I have to accept that. But I have made a commitment to write and I am writing.

When I was at UCLA, transportation planners identified the stages of the elderly as "young old" (sixty-five to seventy-five), "the middle old" (seventy-five to eighty-five) and "old old" (eighty-five and beyond). At the time I was in my late forties and thought those ages distant and remote. Now when I see myself in the category of the elderly, I wince. But again, consistent with my own definition, at least I am "young old." I must still be playing games with myself, although I am trying to move beyond them.

In "Necessary Losses," Judith Viorst writes that in every stage of life one sustains necessary losses, and to grow, one must come to terms with those losses in order to move on to the next stage of growth—and loss.

She writes, "And we may start to feel that this is a time of always letting go, of one thing after another after another: Our waistlines. Our vigor. Our sense of adventure. Our 20/20 vision. Our trust in justice. Our earnestness. Our playfulness. Our dream of being a tennis star, or a senator, or the woman for whom Paul Newman finally leaves Joanne. We give up hoping to read all the books we once had vowed to read, and to go to all of the places we'd once vowed to visit. We give up hoping we'll save the world from cancer or from war. We even give up hoping that we will succeed in becoming underweight—or immortal.

"We feel shaken. We feel scared. We do not feel safe. The center's not holding, and things are falling apart. All of a sudden our friends, if not us, are having affairs, divorces, heart attacks, cancer. Some of our friends—men and women our age—have died. And as we acquire new aches and new pains, our health care is, of necessity, being supplied by internists, cardiologists, dermatologists, podiatrists, urologists, periodontists, gynecologists and psychiatrists, from all of whom we want a second opinion."

She could have been writing about me. No wonder the light went on in my head when I read it.

In a column titled "How Long Do Old Women Have to Be Young?" Ellen Goodman writes "But gradually it has occurred to me that women are only being given an extension on aging. They are not being given permission to age gracefully. The culture is telling women they can be younger longer. It is not welcoming old women."

Need for Identity

In the same way that I yearned and searched for roots, I sought to find my identity. Where had I come from? Who was I?

I had a fierce need for my own identity, to be known as my own person, to accomplish something in life. To be recognized. (To have a byline?) In many ways I was an earlier women's libber, casting my lot with the suffragettes and the early movements towards women's liberation. I carried this ambition forward from childhood into adulthood. And when my first therapist suggested I read Betty Friedan's "The Feminine Mystique," I realized I was not alone in my yearnings. My personal aspirations coalesced with growing attitudes in society: many women wanted to seek recognition outside the home, be valued and measured and rewarded as men were, by their work.

I took for granted that my family was my responsibility and knew there weren't many rewards for raising a family—either with ease or with difficulty. No recognition for a long marriage. These noble activities were diminished in value by society at that time. I must have been influenced by strongly prevailing attitudes toward women, women's place, women's potential. Women's success was being measured by male standards.

How much of women's stress comes from not having the love and care they give their families that count in the world the same way career success counts? Fortunately, society's—and women's—values are changing today to value single mothers, and working women, and women who stay at home, who juggle the conflicting demands on their lives. Even now a shift in attitude toward traditional family values offers promise of recognition for attention to the family.

Even by my own standards, I conceded that I had been successful. Successful in the community, in politics, in the world of work, and in the regard of my colleagues. But when I resigned my position, withdrew from public life and started traveling with Joe, I had come full circle, back to being someone's wife, someone's mother. It wasn't enough for me.

Before My Heart Attack

In the years before the heart attack, I had viewed my life as fragmented, compartmentalized, discontinuous. When I finished high school, I closed off that segment, and didn't carry it forward into college. When I finished college, I left that time and place behind. It was the same when I left politics. And with the American Jewish Committee and UCLA—I slammed the door behind me. They were tidy, discrete, unconnected compartments—or so I thought. The only continuity I felt was with my family.

It wasn't until I lay near death in the hospital that the closed doors were forced open by the floods of affection that came to me from all these former portions of my life, ones that I had so carefully separated. Prayers and letters, books, flowers and calls came from college, political, and work friends. I could not believe that I had such a a host of caring friends. Something had changed in me, although I didn't realize it had been happening for some time: I had begun to value myself as a separate person without public recognition, not a dim shadow in the background. I was sorry it took near death to show me my own value.

After My Heart Attack

The more research I have done on coronary artery disease, the luckier I know I am. I also know about finite time. About the possibility that bypasses do not last forever. That another one, or two, or three arteries could become blocked. That I might not be as lucky the next time. God's plan and benevolence for me may not include another chance.

Yet, I do not want to run around in a frenzy, to jam as much as I can into life; rather I believe I will live as fully and happily as I can, for as long as I am healthy and alive.

Three months after the heart attack I made a resolution to change my life for the sake of my health. Through first-hand research I created my own personal program for recovery and survival. I made my diet an ally, exercise a habit, and stress an entity outside myself. And created a means to keep stress at bay.

I'd like to suggest that you make this resolution before you have to—before heart disease becomes a problem for you, too.

For Good Heart Health:

Don't be afraid of therapy. You're only going to learn and grow. It may be the best investment you make in time and money for preventive medicine.

If you feel stress is an important factor in your life, consider seeing a therapist.

If you see a therapist, bring up the subject of stress.

You can change your attitude about aging. Consider: You are lucky to be alive and growing older.

The younger you are when you discover who you are and what you want, the better your chances are for reducing stress.

Don't judge yourself too harshly.

Modify your schedule and your pace.

You may want to rethink your leisure activities and vacation plans. Remember, the idea is to reduce stress and add pleasure to your life.

The more secure you are about yourself, the easier it is to live with a famous partner, or any partner.

While it may seem strange to think of a heart attack as an inspiration, that's what it became to me.

14. from depression to transformation

During the first months after my recovery, I was undergoing the beginning of a personal transformation, but first I had to get through another unexpected turn. Depression.

Depression always follows bypass surgery, I have learned from University teaching psychiatrists; but they can't convince the cardiac surgeons to tell the patient that this might occur.

I believe this has to change. The doctor has to tell you to expect this as normal part of recovery. The doctor has to tell you about next week, next month, next year, and not just the day after tomorrow. I had wonderful doctors who saved my life, who were very interested in my health and recovery, but never pointed me to the future. As part of the recovery effort, a group of hospital volunteers, patients recovered from heart bypass surgery made an attempt to visit me; I didn't want to see them or any strangers. But if I'd been told by one of my doctors to expect a woman who had experienced what I had, perhaps I would have been more accepting. Maybe we should have support groups for women who have had heart attacks. Best of all, our doctors should tell us about depression, and that being involved with peers will be an important part of our recovery when we return home. If it has the imprimatur of the doctor who has saved us, we'll know it is important and an important part of getting well.

All I saw was a booklet written for the male heart patient with male illustrations and advice for women who take care of the post-surgical male patient. When I read it, I felt left out. Hadn't I, too, a woman, had heart surgery? I'm glad to report that the booklet was revised since I was a patient. Changes such as this make me hopeful. It's one thing to wear men's clothing, it's another to accept a male prototype for what is the marvelous and unique female body.

Women must change how they take care of themselves, and they must campaign for change in treatment from our doctors. We women pushed for natural childbirth, fewer medications, more involvement of the father, and we got it. Now it is accepted as the norm. If women hadn't insisted on change, we wouldn't now have deliveries where husband and families participate. If women would now do what they did in childbirth, we could transform treatment for heart disease. Even though the majority of women experience heart disease when they're older, I think they could mount an intelligent, vigorous, rational campaign to turn things around.

It would have been helpful for me to know that my daily weeping was to be expected. That my unnatural inclination to curl up in bed and not push myself was part of my post operative depression. In some way, I coupled it with the awe of the experience I was being told about. But I was depressed, emotional, and I was not sure of anything, especially that I would ever get well. I cried every day, when a gift came, when a letter came, when flowers came, when I learned who had been calling Joe at home and how helpful our friends had been to him.

When the nurse asked me to start doing more for myself, I resisted; I was afraid to stand. And when I took my first steps to the bathroom, I felt as if I were walking on the thin shaky legs of my mother-in-law, rather than my ample limbs. Every first step I took, I was afraid. It continued well into my recovery.

Near the end of my three week hospital stay, I began to face the enormity of what I'd been through. I was frightened. When I came home I was facing my dying and coming back; what did it mean and feel like? Frightened again, and angry, too, that this could have happened to me, and that I had to face the reality that I was not entirely in control of my life. I idealized Carlos as my savior, and somehow this was a thread-like lifeline that began to pull me through the depression

Making The Best Use of Rehabilitation

When I got home, the first person I called for, other than family, was my psychiatrist. She came to my bedside as I cried and poured out my fear, anxiety, depression and growing awareness of my ordeal. I don't think I could have made it without her help.

Although I hated it and was frightened of it at first, the rehabilitation was another important payoff for me. The physical exercise was combating the depression, although I did not realize its impact at the time.

When I went to cardiac rehabilitation thirteen days after release from the hospital, I was afraid to step on the treadmill. When I heard my heart pounding, resonating in my chest, I could not distinguish between a normal heart sound and the echo chamber I sensed. When I had pains in my back, I was sure that I was having another heart attack.

When Joe tried to persuade me I was strong enough to go out of town five weeks after my dismissal from the hospital, I objected, but just to please him (my historic pattern) and full of apprehension, I agreed to go to a meeting in Napa, and afterward to the wedding of my sister-in-law's son near San Francisco. I rested a great deal, but I also gained a tiny bit of confidence, though I couldn't see it at the time. As we walked along the seaside path, a cold stiff wind blew up, almost knocking me down, and I was frightened that I'd be blown back to Cedars-Sinai. I turned my back to the gale, huddled against Joe and somehow we got into the corner of a building till it subsided. My heart was racing, and my chest hurt. But this activity, too, was a depression fighter.

Strengthening Ties to Family and Friends

A sea change came in my relationship with Edna and David, my son and daughter-in-law. They came to say they were reconsidering their decision to move back to Israel because of what had happened to me. For the five years they lived in California after returning from Israel, they had felt frustrated about the amount of time we spent together, attributing it to our lack of desire and interest rather than the pressure of juggling their schedules and ours, of traffic and complexity of living in Los Angeles, as well as the travels and demands placed on us by Joe's public life. Now they saw that their parents could become endangered species, taken away from them in a flash; now they were rethinking the importance of family relationships. When they brought this up at my bedside, I said to them, as I had five years before, "You have to go; you have to do what is best for you."

Edna came to share her most intimate thoughts and secrets, to ask advice, the first time she had ever done so in their marriage. And I cried and cried. I don't know what that was; but a heightened sensitivity, reactive emotionalism set in. These were not sad tears, but tears of growth, wonder, awe, tears of love.

Fred, the eldest and most tender-hearted of my children, was at Joe's side and mine throughout the ordeal. He wanted to give his blood back to me, the source from whence it came.

I think his devotion was an impetus for me to recover, to reassure him.

Sarah, with a congenital heart condition, was the most stoical of the family. Now she and I both had imperfect (damaged) hearts.

Joe was the cheerleader. He never showed me any fear or doubt. He says he always believed in my recovery and that's what he passed on to me.

By the time mother died, I realized I was neither depressed nor anxious. I was sad, not disabled, and I was getting well. By late May or early June, the depression was under control. Had I been keeping a depression diary, my notations would have begun in March and ended in June. And I did it through my own efforts.

Not only did my relationship with my children change but also with my stylish, beautiful and much younger-than-I, sister-in-law Nancy. We loved each other, but in a distant, tightly reserved manner, we broke through to a new level of devotion. "What if I had lost you and I hadn't ever told you how I felt?" she said.

She came to talk, to bring me things, to offer any assistance. I accepted and turned to her for help many times during my recovery.

At that time I did not know how powerful love is as a healing factor. Medical research shows that love, hope, faith and laughter are well-known sources of strength and healing.

Within weeks after I came home, my mother-in-law died. I was still too weak to attend her funeral and pay her my last loving respects, and this kicked up the depression again, but deep down, I promised to push myself toward recovery. I wanted to see my mother again, and as often as I could.

Luckily, I was soon allowed to drive and visit her almost daily, as I had before my heart attack. Except that it cheered her when I was there, I am not sure it made a difference, and I know she did not remember after I left. That's the way it had been for many, many months. Three months after my heart surgery, Mother collapsed at home and was rushed to the hospital, probably already dead. When the emergency physician called to say mother was dead, I told Joe I wanted to go to the hospital to see her. He said he didn't think it was a good idea.

"Honey, I'm going to go. You don't have to go in with me. Either you can drive me or I will drive myself," I said.

"I'll take you, Mickey," he said.

Now I had buried both my parents, one in the fullness of his life, the other having existed beyond her definition of living. I took charge of breaking up Mother's household, with some help from my siblings. And I went home to grieve and to remember and to keep her presence and wisdom in me. I think of her every day. Many things about my mother are in me, but lately, as I think about my close, warm affectionate relationship with my doctors, I think of my mother, who had profound respect, dependence, great attachment, and at the end, an almost child-like gratitude to her doctors.

My mother's death reconfirmed my resolution to use my experience to improve my life. I had decided to allow my heart attack to change my whole way of life, and the only way to do this was to make heart disease a positive ally, to look at it as an opportunity for change. While it may seem strange to think of a heart attack as an inspiration, it is the only way to go.

I allowed the near death experience to transform my life. A sense of connectedness crept in and it has permeated my life and fertilized my future, inspiring me to live a whole life. I had kept contentment away by denying that any of my prior life's experiences had any connection to the next one.

Many things have happened to me that would not have happened had I not had a heart attack and nearly died. I have come to appreciate living every day, even though I forget some time. I have come closer to my family, now able to relate to my children as adults. And my sister and I have become close friends. Not a week goes by without our talking long distance several times. We took a vacation together to Texas to visit friends, something I would not have thought of doing before, just going off on a trip without Joe.

I had experienced an emotional catharsis that I was almost unaware of—maybe it was the same lack of awareness that I had about my heart disease before the heart attack.

I was able to jump back in time, hurtling over the pain of the suicide to remember pleasant moments with my father. I remember Daddy being proud of me as a child, teaching me about business, taking me with him to make bank deposits, to the post office to help handle business mail, teaching me about insurance and contracts, to read every line of a form before I signed it, teaching me how to open his safe. When I received the American Legion award in high school, he beamed with pride in his first-born child, a full-fledged and honored American.

After Joe's Mother died, his father slipped into senility, but occasional flashes of his basic personality shone through. He remained stubborn, physically strong and strong-willed almost to the end. Once after he fell on the sloping driveway at his house, the paramedics could hardly wrestle him onto a gurney and into the ambulance. Otherwise, he was in excellent health, yet terribly sad, depressed and confused because he knew something was wrong with him, that he couldn't remember things, didn't know where he was, didn't know exactly what had happened to him. I had learned this behavior watching my mother fail.

Now, sympathy and empathy made it easy to relate to my father-in-law, to talk to him, to repeat stories and answer his repeated question, and sometimes, to get him to remember incidents from earlier days when he was a pioneer in Los Angeles. My old feelings changed, and when he died, I was shocked at how grief-stricken and upset I was.

Reunion and Deliverance

I wanted to go back to Texas, to my roots. I went back home for my 50th high school reunion. As Joe and I drove the streets and country roads around Mercedes, I experienced a completely unexpected mystic return to the geography, to the land. I took possession of my past—the person I was and the place I was born. The flat landscape, acres of freshly plowed earth, bright-green growing crops, and pure blue skies filled with billowing mountains of clouds reminded me of my childhood, and pulled me back into connection.

I came with my sister Berty (whose class joined mine in reunion), and with Joe, to share this experience with him, and to share him with the picture-taking and autograph-seeking fans from my graduating class.

I found something else special. My high school boyfriend, W.B. "Dub" Lauder, had been in a near fatal automobile accident three months earlier. He waved aside most inquiries into his condition with a smile on his face and full of denial, saying "It was all a mistake, it didn't happen." On the outside, he looked well and whole, brown hair gone gray, still slender, still running, still connected to life. But he had lain unconscious for many weeks, hooked up to tubes and trying like a wild man to pull them out as his wife, Jean, kept a bedside vigil.

Fifty years fell away. It was more than two old folks sharing medical stories of crisis, survival and transformation. Two old friends, miraculously saved, helping each other understand about our lives.

"Dub, your story with Jean is like mine with Joe. Have you told her how much it meant to you for her to be there?" I asked.

"No, I really don't think so. It's really hard for me," he said.

"I can't seem to get the words out. As soon as I got well, I went back to work. I started pushing the way I had before."

"You've got to stop denying what happened to you," I said. "You had this second chance, just like I did. Make the most of it!"

It was a brief encounter, measured in the stream of life, but important and deeply meaningful to both of us, probably something we will always remember. I am haunted by the intensity of the emotion, of an eerie transcendence, of how, worlds apart, not really knowing each other after all these years, we were able to speak as mature friends who had shared a miracle.

Solving the mystery of my daughter's birth was a way of taking charge of my life.

15. an awakening

There have been many bonuses to my experience, new ways of looking at life, valuing friends and family, making connections, reconnecting. But one awakening came unexpectedly: in a casual disagreement with Joe.

I said, "I'm indebted to Cedars for saving my life twice—once just now, and once when Sarah was born and I was in a coma for ten days."

"You weren't in a coma for ten days," he said, giving me no room to disagree, as usual.

Here was a situation that used to make me feel out of control. Now, I could let the remark pass, take charge and control. That's just what I did.

In an instant I knew that I wouldn't argue with Joe, that I would seek other avenues to confirm my memory. After all these years I still wanted to know what had happened the night Sarah was born. The obstetrician was dead. The pediatrician was dead. My Bill Molle didn't remember, but said he didn't think I had been comatose ten days. Not satisfied, I called Cedars-Sinai. No, they did not keep records from 1958.

I set out to solve a mystery. Solving this mystery was a different way of taking charge of my life. It seemed as if I were trying to weave the disparate threads of my life into one whole tapestry. Remaining for me was a source I had etched indelibly on my mind: Dr. Walter Fox, the young, on-duty senior resident obstetrician who saved my life at Cedars of Lebanon many years ago. I wondered if he was still in practice, still in Los Angeles. When I called his office, he came on the phone immediately and said, "What happened to you? You told me when I came back from the army, you would become my patient." Yes, he remembered me; yes, he remembered the case, yes; I could come to talk to him.

Not only did Dr. Fox remember, but so did Connie Czarnetski, his office nurse, who had been on duty in the delivery room the night Sarah was born.

"I've come to ask you to help me find out what happened to me and Sarah the night she was born," I said.

"You were in room 56, the private room near the nursing station," Connie said. "I remember zooming down the hall to get magnesium sulfate, which we gave for toxemia at delivery."

My mouth fell open. I shook my head in disbelief.

Dr. Fox picked up the story. "You had elevated blood pressure, probably albumen. You had a convulsion not too long after delivery. You had had an anesthetic caudal. In 1958 they were using two-percent zylocaine and sometimes to fill up the caudal space, they put in a sizable dose of medication."

When Dr. Fox was called in to see me about the convulsion, he said he gave me phenobarbital intravenously, sedated me and after that there were no further episodes.

I looked from Connie to Dr. Fox. "How could you remember all that after more than thirty years?" I said.

"I followed you. I took an interest in your case since you felt that you'd been saved. I felt more involved." he said.

Dr. Fox said that I was not allowed to nurse Sarah because of the phenobarbital in my system and concern that something else might happen while I was holding the baby.

"The reason I've been so certain about the ten days coma all these years is that I remember a nurse asking me to go on a bedpan and I told her I couldn't do it," I said. 'What do you think you've been doing for the past ten days?' the nurse asked me."

"But I know for sure you were not comatose for ten days, maybe ten to fifteen minutes," he said.

"It was because of the fairly large dose of medication we gave you that you wouldn't have any recollection of what happened. You might have been dreaming," he said. "You had a total lack of recall, amnesia for the event, no independent recollection of what transpired. For all intents and purposes you were not there," Dr. Fox said.

I fell silent, taking it all in. Now I knew about the delivery night, but I had more long-festering questions.

I told Dr. Fox that for the thirty-three years since that day, I had needed to make connections between Sarah's developmental inconsistencies, her early maladroitness, her aortic stenosis, her learning difficulties and the toxemia I was convinced I had suffered during my entire pregnancy.

"I have always believed toxemia was the cause of it all, although I could never get a doctor to say so," I said.

"No," Dr. Fox said, "Your toxemia didn't carry all through pregnancy. Yours is a misperception. Your toxemia was acute. What you had was intrauterine growth retardation, where the placenta is not healthy enough to support a fully grown child."

"Instead of the child being nourished at the maximum that a normal placenta does," he went on, "your placenta had infarcts in it and it had a diminution of the ability to transfer oxygen to the infant. What happens is that growth is inhibited. Sometimes there are growth inhibitions that are also involved with mentation, cerebration, because the brain has to be nourished also."

Tears welled up in my eyes and fell over my face. He was giving me the missing link. The stone came off my shoulders. Freedom.

"It is impossible to actually reconstruct what was going on intrauterine with you at the time, but we know something must have been going on," Dr. Fox said. "The fact that she was small and delivered at full term or near full term is a clue."

I asked Dr. Fox if things had changed since then.

"In today's world you would be able to examine the placenta, the size of the child and relate it and sometimes deliver babies prematurely because the environment inside the uterus is hostile," he said. "But she was born in an era before ultrasound, biophysical profiles, in an era before we were able to know these things. That's the way it was. The best obstetricians at the time would not have delivered prematurely. At that time we let the baby grow in the uterus, waited and hoped they'd live long enough in the uterus to get big enough to be delivered. We were short on information at that time.

"What you had was an accident of nature in the way the placenta evolved. We know more about it now, what to do about it, but we still don't have any good explanation about why it happens."

And then he answered a question that had been nagging me for years. "It was nothing you did or didn't do, or anything Dr. B. did or didn't do. There is nothing he could have done earlier that would have made any difference. Nothing he could have done that would have changed the co-arctation of the aorta. That is a congenital, incorrect evolution of the process that's supposed to have taken place in that area."

I was crying and trying to thank him, but he wouldn't let me go before I promised to listen to his advice.

"You need to give yourself a pat on the back for all you've done and stop worrying about what you have not done," he said. "It seems reasonable you've agonized a great deal. You've done a lot, thought a lot, been as helpful as humanly possible. But you can't go beyond this. Learn to forgive yourself again and again and again. Be easier on yourself. There weren't any resources at the time."

Now I knew. I was stunned and silent. Exhausted, relieved,

overwhelmed with what I had learned. And somehow, at peace. I had found the missing piece of the puzzle that had dominated the last thirty-three years of my life.

Joe was quiet and pensive when I told him. "So now we know," he said.

I could not go back and rewrite history; I could not change Sarah's life or mine, erase the psychological scars left on both of us for not knowing. But I could share this new information with her and reassert that I had done the best I could with what I knew. She didn't seem as relieved as I; her life had not been as great a mystery to her as it had been to me. We came to yet a higher plateau of understanding and insight, and now *she* owns all the knowledge of her development.

I could not have known about this had I not had the heart attack. I could not have received this deliverance had I not had cardiac arrest and the subsequent crisis, and the motivation to explore my life's stresses. I could not have discovered this truth had I not wanted to thank God and Cedars-Sinai for saving my life twice.

Part Four

Blockage of the arteries is a linear process that starts early; women who aren't careful at a young age are likely to start at a disadvantage when the risks of menopause take hold.

16. what I learned from my heart attack

I have learned to love life so passionately that I want to do everything in my power to stay healthy, to live as long and as happily as I can. I've learned a lot about heart disease. and heart disease in women. And stress. My life's passion today is to share my experience and knowledge, to help others stay alive, get well, stay well. Some things that I have learned for myself are what I'd like to share.

Prevention and Preparedness

At the outset I would like to make a radical proposal: that every woman over fifty have a consultation with a cardiologist and a stress test. This is the right time to establish a baseline reading on your heart health, your cholesterol reading and your blood pressure. Thereafter, schedule regular check-ups with your cardiologist or your internist to give you a road map about how your heart is functioning. This should create an atmosphere for further on-going discussion about your risks for heart disease. I never had that stress test. Heart disease can be simply hereditary and a stress test will detect heart disease no matter what its source. I make this recommendation in the face of a changing and uncertain future for medical practice, insurance availability and general support for health care. But I say it anyway; I look upon this as the highest level of self-protection.

Every day I hear women in their early fifties and into their sixties say they are experiencing back pain, a little pressure in the chest, a little indigestion. "It will go away. It's nothing." They could be having a heart attack. And what do we do? We deny. We delay. I would like to scream.

I'm screaming now. TAKE CARE OF YOURSELVES.

I have learned to take charge of my life; that doesn't mean I choose every activity, but I never do anything I can't accept or be comfortable with.

The first line of defense is to have a good doctor in your life, a smart one, who listens to you, one you trust, and one who understands a woman's unique medical circumstances. If you get the run-around, find yourself being patronized, your symptoms ignored, change doctors immediately.

I have probably the best cardiologist in the city—and I'm sensitizing him to women's heart disease. Since there's so little research—and he's a researcher in arrhythmias—I'm glad he's listening.

Develop an emergency plan for yourself. After all, you've done it for your kids. Write the plan, give copies to family and neighbors, post it by the phone.

Identify the closest top level emergency hospital—one where you could go for a heart attack—not to sew up a cut hand or set a broken bone—and think about the fastest way to get there. If you are experiencing chest pain, shortness of breath, calling an ambulance is a good idea. You'll get life saving attention on the way to the emergency room. If you call 911, you will receive emergency assistance on the spot, and they will contact your doctor, but they are required to take you to the nearest emergency facility, and that may not be where you ought to go. If the doctor is in your life, he or she will be the first one you call in an emergency, and the doctor will direct your emergency care.

At the very first sign of chest pain or suspicious symptoms, call the doctor; get yourself to the emergency room. Don't be stoical. Don't wait. Go. Every minute is precious. Doctors I know prefer to bundle their family emergency patients into their own cars and drive to the hospital as fast as they can. And don't worry if its a false alarm. Men go to the hospital for chest pains that turn out to be indigestion, without thinking twice.

Things we can do to take care of ourselves bear repeating:

STOP SMOKING, if you smoke. There are many programs designed to help smokers stop—at hospitals, churches and synagogues, local health facilities, commercial programs. There is no question, smoking is the number one health hazard.

LOWER YOUR CHOLESTEROL LEVEL: Recent findings suggest we should be watching what our children eat from the age of two, so as to reduce the long, slow build-up of plaque in the arteries. This is no mystery; a diet low in fat—without meat, dairy products and eggs—in combination with an exercise program works. Dean Ornish has demonstrated that such a program can reverse cholesterol levels, reduce plaque, help a patient avoid surgery. A strict vegetarian diet is the most dramatic and significant way to accomplish this reduction. Your doctor, the American Heart Association, and "how to" books on heart disease can give you these guidelines.

AVOID OBESITY: Lose weight and keep it off. What you do to lower cholesterol usually results in achieving and maintaining the recommended body weight.

EXERCISE: A brisk thirty-minute walk five-to-seven times a week will do wonders for your psyche, increase stamina, relieve stress, reduce cholesterol levels—and tone your body. Some like to join exercise programs at their churches or the Y or a program connected with a cardiac prevention center at the local hospital. It is important to have a physical check-up first, commence exercising gradually and increase the level so that you are receiving optimum benefits, but not pushing beyond safety. And it is important to find something you like to do and stick to it.

CONTROL ALCOHOL, CAFFEINE AND DRUGS: If you're involved with any of these addictive substances, get tough with yourself. Be disciplined. Don't make excuses. Reduce and limit your intake of alcohol and caffeine. Try to give them up entirely. And drugs have no place in the life of a healthy individual. Kick the habit; get help to do it.

In Consultation with Your Doctor, Consider Also:

HORMONE REPLACEMENT THERAPY, if you are post menopausal. I am keen on this therapy. The natural protection women enjoy before menopause disappears after its onset. Although there are frequent contradictory reports in the popular press, there is general agreement that hormone replacement therapy reduces the risk of heart disease, is a protection against osteoporosis (brittle, breakable bones especially in elderly women), and a possible protection against some cancers.

I eavesdrop in elevators, at pharmacy counters, wherever I am and especially when women are talking about hormone replacement therapies. It takes a lot of restraint to keep from entering those conversations, but fortunately most of them end well.

ASPIRIN: Research has shown that half an aspirin, two times a day, has demonstrated equal value for women and men and it needs to be taken.

VITAMINS: Adding large doses of vitamins C, E and Beta Carotene which act as anti-oxidants to reduce risk of heart disease.

PSYLLIUM, a natural fiber, good for regulating bowels and thought to help roll away dietary fats in the process.

SCREENING: Be aware of the tests that are available for diagnosing heart disease. And if you think or know you are at risk for heart disease, explore the possibility of screening and test options with your doctors. I want women to be as aware of tests for heart disease as they are of the pap smear to detect cancer.

I'm beginning to think that our best bet is to have skillfully trained, sensitive and aware OB-Gyns and all primary care physicians involved in our heart histories. They are the ones we know best, whom we relate to. They know us best. Maybe they will be the ones to teach the internists and cardiologists to pay attention to women.

What are we to do about apparently conflicting studies about what to eat and what not to eat, how to exercise, whether to pay attention to cholesterol or not? Most scientists have urged a lower cholesterol level—under 200, and now comes a study that says "high cholesterol is less risky for the elderly." Who and what are we to believe? Rather than ping-ponging about from one study to another, and taking matters into our own hands, we must take these reports to our doctors and let them sort them out for us. We need our doctor's input and guidance before we change any course of treatment. I, personally, will opt for a moderate life style and diet, and a regular stepped-up exercise program. Moderation feels right for me.

REDUCE STRESS: I have purposely left this for last, because it is the most complex and least objective of the recommendations. Again, many self-help books give suggestions and programs for learning to manage stress; many of them are helpful. The necessary first step is to determine what causes your stress, and how you react to it. That's going to require taking a hard look into yourself and asking yourself questions—like how and where, and when and with whom, you experience stress, perhaps seeking professional help in the process. You might keep a diary and jot down circumstances that cause your stress.

Most medical schools' psychiatry departments have an anxiety or stress clinic where they do evaluations and help people see what their sources of stress are. Standard techniques are often used for relaxation training, cognitive restructuring and developing planning skills.

If the nature of the stress is extreme, like the death of a spouse at the same time that the individual is caring for an aging parent, that kind of severe stress may require intense psychotherapy and utilization of support systems.

And lots of organizations provide stress counseling.

MEDITATION: Several methods of meditation, which require a minimum of instruction and practice, performed for just twenty minutes twice a day, or used to interrupt a stressful situation, can bring inner peace. A good book or a friend who meditates can teach you. I describe the method I learned in the next section.

BIOFEEDBACK: This assisted stress management method uses sensitive technology to record physiological factors; a patient is made aware of his or her emotional responses; follow-up techniques, such as meditation, are recommended.

I don't look at any of these as a burden, but as an opportunity to take care of myself, promote good health and prolong my life. Looking at it this way, there's no sacrifice. The lifestyle change is a "pepper-upper."

Rehabilitation

Just as a heart attack changes your life forever, cardiac rehabilitation can push you back to living. It gave me courage and taught me how to care for and heal myself. Other recovering patients give the same testimony. While I entered the program a skeptic, I graduated a booster.

My cardiac rehabilitation began in my hospital bed with simple supervised painful body movements and graduated to hospital corridor walks by the time of discharge. The staff sent me home with a list of daily exercises to perform for the few weeks before I entered their three-month cardiac rehabilitation program.

Where to Go for Help

In every major city where there are academic research centers connected with cardiac surgery programs, there are likely to be follow-up therapy programs. Most community and private hospitals also sponsor rehab programs. Unfortunately, there are no licensing procedures to credential the good ones or to weed out the inferior ones. You'll want to look for something connected with a reputable institution. And you'll want to make sure the personnel are well-trained, that the overall program is prescribed after you pass a medical exam, that you are carefully monitored by staff and equipment. Most treatment programs are covered by insurance. Again, ask your doctor. If he or she is casual or indifferent about it, don't take the easy way out; insist that you be given a prescription/referral to the program. Go!

You and your doctor will be happy with your recovery.

For approximately twelve weeks you will work with a team of doctors, nurses, exercise physiologists, psychologists and dietitians to modify your lifestyle that will progressively rebuild your strength, endurance and confidence.

Most centers require a patient to take a stress test prior to enrolling and to forward medical records as reference for the rehab team. Then a patient is interviewed and carefully evaluated. You will be given a lengthy questionnaire, and asked for previous medical history, symptoms of heart disease, specific events accompanying the heart attack, treatment and/or surgery. You will have an interview and questionnaire with the consulting psychologist to ascertain need and formulate a personal stress management program. Some programs use scientific measurements to precisely record stress in a simulated life situation. Finally, you will have an introduction to the use of the variety of machines in the exercise program.

The day Joe took me in for this initial appointment, I wanted to run away. What could they tell me about cooking and lowering cholesterol that I didn't know? What could the psychologist tell me when I already had a psychiatrist? I hated the exercise bicycle (I had owned one and given it away.) The treadmill scared me. Why couldn't I just go back to walking? I learned.

Programs vary, of course, but basically they consist of a number of equally important parts:

Careful screening and evaluation.
Education about the cardiovascular system, risk factors for
   heart disease.
Stress, anger, and anxiety management.
Eating to lower blood cholesterol—eating at home, and
   finding healthy options in supermarket and restaurant.
A structured, progressive, monitored exercise program.

In addition most centers make available personal, private consultations to further deal with nutrition, stress reduction, psychological needs, referrals for genetic testing, special programs for diabetics, biofeedback programs. Support groups also advance the rehab process.

Very sick patients, some whose recovery is unsatisfactory, slow and difficult, require the services of highly specialized programs applying the latest research. Consultation with your doctor to identify these major centers is a must—not to be postponed.

Young women stand poised on the brink of an epidemic of stress-related diseases, including heart disease.

17. what's in store for the next generation

If stress plays as large a role in the development of heart disease as many experts now believe, what's to become of the baby-boom generation of women?

The first of the boomers are now turning fifty, the menopausal point in life at which their heart-disease risk begins its ascent. They are products of the post-1950's work-outside-the-home surge in which working women became the norm rather than the exception.

So women began working in record numbers: 23 million in 1960, 32 million in 1970, 45 million in 1980, 58 million today. Naysayers warned that the prize for taking on the professional trappings of men would be their stress-related diseases. They forgot something: women have other pressures to deal with as well.

American women—even those who work—still bear the brunt of child-rearing, still do most of the cooking and cleaning, and still do the majority of the caring for elderly parents or parents-in-law who need assistance. A 1989 study of professionals at a Swedish car-manufacturing plant found that when male managers got home after a day's work, their blood pressure dropped immediately. Female managers, on the other hand, failed to unwind until much later in the evening.

Life in our fast-paced society seems to become more stressful every day. The American Academy of Family Physicians now estimates that two-thirds of office visits to family doctors are stress-related.

Meanwhile, women's average life expectancy is now 79, fully one-third of it after menopause. With everyone living longer, women, whose heart-disease symptoms begin at a later age, are at higher risk. And aging itself brings on many sources of stress—the loss of loved ones, loss of status, decreased mobility, financial difficulties, ill health, and new living arrangements, to name a few.

All of which beg the question: Will we see an explosion of stress-related heart disease in the next generation of women?

The answer is unclear. Because of varying definitions of stress, research has produced conflicting results. Some studies have shown more stress in women working outside the home; others suggest that staying at home in a society that devalues housework can lower self-esteem and create stress of its own. Some indicate that women executives in high-pressure professions suffer the most; others find blue-collar or middle-management jobs, in which woman have less control over their daily duties and less money to dole out on child-care, take the greatest toll. Common sense dictates that juggling multiple roles produces stress, but many studies have found that the more roles a woman balances, the more psychologically healthy she is.

"A lot of people feel that women taking on multiple roles is actually beneficial, that it gives them different sources of satisfaction and self-esteem," notes Dr. Karen Matthews, a professor of psychiatry at the University of Pittsburgh School of Medicine who has studied physiological responses to stress and found that the magnitude of women's stress responses increases after menopause.

Matthews points out that the stresses experienced by women might be more interpersonal than job-related, that family and relationship troubles are often more of a factor than work-related issues.

In an attempt to determine whether professional women "would look more like men" in terms of stress-related illnesses, Matthews has followed a group of high-level federal employees for more than a decade and found little evidence to support her hypothesis.

But this was a group of women with a solid income and no risk of losing their jobs, Matthews notes. "If we had studied a less-extreme group, we might have had a different picture."

"Maybe we haven't done the right research," says Dr. Bairey Merz. "Or maybe the hypothesis is wrong."

Or maybe, since women develop heart disease later in life than the age of this generation's oldest members, we can't know yet? Are these women old enough that we could even say?

Just as I was a pioneer for my generation, juggling multiple roles as wife, mother, social activist, and professional, then subsequently experiencing heart disease, the next generation of young women, now in their late forties and early fifties, may stand poised on the brink of an epidemic of stress-related diseases, including heart disease.

I care very much about this next generation of younger women—my daughters, my nieces, my sisters—coming up after me. These young pioneers who have charted new paths for themselves in work, in family relationships, in parenting, need to pay attention, to take a moment to stop racing and juggling and creating and problem solving. Take a moment to stand still, to take stock, to care for themselves and about themselves.

Today's most popular buzz words are stress and exercise.

What's clear is that these pioneering boomers need to take care of themselves. I believe that while they have been charged with being the most narcissistic of generations, they can turn it

YEAR	WOMEN IN THE WORK FORCE	% OF WOMEN WORKING
1960	23,240,000	37.7
1970	31,543,000	43.3
1980	45,487,000	51.5
1990	56,554,000	57.5
1992	57,798,000	57.8
2005*	75,394,000	63.0

*Projected.

Source: U.S. Dept. of Labor, Women's Bureau (Mike Williams)

NUMBER OF WOMEN MAINTAINING FAMILIES (SINGLE-PARENT):

  1980: 10,582,000

  1986: 11,328,000

  1993: 12,494,000

Source: U.S. Dept. of Labor, Women's Bureau (Mike Williams)

NUMBER OF WOMEN TURNING 50:

  1990: 1,325,000

  1992: 1,592,000

  PROJECTED:

  2000: 1,972,000

  2010: 2,410,000

  2020: 2,165,000

Source: U.S. Bureau of Census, Population Division

around to save their own lives. They can turn around the statistics on women dying of heart disease if they can mount campaigns to insist upon more research on women and heart disease.

They can now face menopause with the openness they've brought to sexuality and sexual relations.

They can fill another gap by urging that more research is needed on the cycle of hormones as a part of a woman's life. Does a valium give on the first day of the hormonal cycle have the same effect as on the sixth? They can urge research by the patriarchal medical profession which has not studied the female heart *as a female heart.* According to Dr. Marianne L. Legato, women's and men's EKG tracings reveal different timing of a portion of the electrical complex, with hormones probably playing a role.

By the time she's forty a woman should have an electrocardiogram (EKG) every year as part of her complete physical, screening test to determine blood cholesterol, and a complete blood lipid profile to determine her triglycerides and HDL/LDL breakdown. Some doctors are recommending stress tests for women as early as thirty-five to forty-five. I wish I had had one.

What I do — What I recommend

I walk a brisk forty minutes a day at a progressively more difficult incline on the treadmill, stretching before and after my workout. I have added a few weight bearing exercises.

I have completely changed my diet: chicken, turkey, and fish, lots of pasta, fresh fruits and vegetables, no meat.

I do not drink because of an unexpected hospitalization for a bout of pancreatitis.

I take Mevacor to reduce my cholesterol level (now usually between 165 and 178, with good relationships between HDL/LDL, and triglycerides). I take baby aspirin two times a day to thin my blood, and Vitamin C, Vitamin E and Beta-Carotene. My doctors believe in hormone replacement therapy, so I take both premarin and progestin.

I try to follow the advice that I learned in cardiac rehab.— I meditate. I sit in a darkened room in a comfortable chair. I progressively contract and relax my eyes, mouth, shoulders, arms, hands, stomach, legs and feet. Then I begin a rhythmic repetition of my chosen words (a prayer) and at the same time visualize a relaxing scene (usually rushing rapids in a river, or a pastoral country scene I remember from England), and breathe regularly and deeply. After twenty minutes, I am refreshed. It is better than a nap some days. And when I feel anger, stress or anxiety coming, meditation aborts them. When I can't sleep at night, I start to repeat my meditation and drift off. My instructor taught me to use the meditation phrase when I am stuck in traffic or find myself in a stressful setting. It works for me.

If I get angry, I let it go. I've learned to ascertain my needs and act upon them, usually in a quiet, reasoned and firm manner.

I'm trying to learn to play, to schedule pleasurable activities.

I've organized my home and workplace. I feel in control.

I never look for things I've misplaced. They always turn up. Saves me time and wear and tear.

I don't take shit. (I couldn't have said that before.)

I am grateful for the opportunity to have experienced life from another perspective, to have learned—through friendship, through stress and success—how to view life with humor and curiosity and skepticism.

I had a spiritual transformation and I wanted to know what had really happened during those dark hours after my bypass surgery. Why had I been chosen to survive?

18. conclusion

Before my heart attack, I believed that as I closed one chapter in my life and moved into another, I had shut the door, closing out the past, obliterating it, giving it no relevance to the present. Afterward I learned how continuous the strand of life is even as it is tenuous. I learned the power of love and the power of prayer, and I truly could not separate one from the other. I knew that power beyond the walls of Cedars-Sinai had played a part in my recovery.

Much has been written about deathbed conversions to another faith, deathbed return to God. That assumes a level of consciousness which I do not think I possessed when these thoughts and feelings fluttered and then surged into my awareness. I had struggled with the god concept at both a religious and intellectual level for most of my adult life, never coming to terms with the question, never being able to suspend my disbelief, not being willing to abandon entirely periods of agnosticism or of atheism.

But as I lay in my bed recovering, waves of gratitude swept over me: thankfulness to Carlos and to John, to Bill and Harold, to Cedars-Sinai, to my family's faith and love and prayers, and for something beyond all of that, and beyond all of my previous experience, I was thankful to God. I felt that the admitting team in the Emergency Room on the morning of admission had been angels, surrounding me, carrying me to survival. That both John and Carlos were God's agents working miracles through their gifted work and hands. Why else would they have worked so hard and so long beyond normal procedures to save me?

I knew that I had had a transformative experience. I made no pledges to myself, except that I found myself less judgmental and more patient, discovered that I was more accepting of peoples' differences. Once a fiercely independent woman, I was now able to accept a level of dependence, even interdependence. My vulnerability had chastened me, and I felt blessed and not threatened by death. Wonder and awe seemed to become permanent companions.

Joe told me what had happened, Bill told me, Carlos told me. Little by little it began to sink in, even as the specialists came and went. I could not know, I did not know and, now, I still do not know how I survived. But why should I have had any special insight when the doctors did not? I have felt a sense of awe and wonder in nature, in special beautiful places in the world, at a sunrise, a sunset, in the touch and smile and embrace of my children and husband, at some natural phenomenon, either positive or negative, even in the fury of disasters, and I have accepted them as cause and effect, the natural order. Because of what I learned and what I felt, I knew there was something more.

When I spoke to my doctors about the operation, the cardiac arrest, the crisis and my recovery, they unanimously felt that something beyond their medical practices had been at work. Bill Molle said that the "Good Lord was looking after you. It really was a miracle, if you talk of medical miracles."

Carlos said, "It was quite an experience for all of us, for everybody, not only for me. Everybody remembers, they know exactly what happened. It's like a miracle."

I told him that because of what happened I had become a believing person, that I was not before.

"I think this became a lesson not only for you, but for everybody. It goes beyond science, it goes beyond life," he said.

Carlos told me that as long as he lived he would remember my case as the one that taught him the most about life and about "our human limitations, our poor understanding about how the body works."

Harold Marcus tends to be fatalistic. He agreed that part of it was a lot of expert and dedicated medical people, but even when they apply the highest level of skill and attention, the patient dies, while at other times when something has been done grossly incorrectly, the outcome turns out to be very good.

"So you can't help but believe that from time to time there is something more, over and above the things that are readily apparent, whatever you want to call it without being religious," he said.

During a post-surgery examination, Jack Matloff and I spoke about my crisis. I was brimming with gratitude, attributing my survival to his team. Jack shook his head, pointed heavenward and said, "He saved your life."

Later, when we talked at length, he said, "I believe there is something far beyond what we as humans do while we're here. If there is something more, something beyond the science of medicine, even biologic science in its greater context that determines these issues. So, for me, arriving at a religious perception of life has been a matter of looking at the facts and accepting them."

"Something happened to me while I was here that hadn't happened anywhere else, a life-affirming experience that has given me a lot of peace," I said.

"You had this experience. You were obviously chosen to be a survivor," he said.

Mickey's Tips

For women of my generation and the next, learning to handle stress must be a primary goal when we look at our overall health and risk for heart disease. There are simple changes in behavior—simple, but not easy—that may prove helpful:

- Have a confidant/friend/minister/counselor or therapist to talk to.
- Practice self-talks, positive, constructive ones that analyze and decrease hostile responses to troublesome situations.
- Learn to laugh, find humor in a situation.
- Avoid an event, place or person.
- Plan how to deal with stress.
- Forgive and forget.
- Learn to express your needs and feeling in a calm, clear, fair way.
- Listen.
- Plan a pleasant activity every day; learn to play.
- Be around pleasant people.
- Take charge of your life. Organize your home, your workspace.

Don't take shit from anyone. (Here I go again.)

None of this is easy. Newly learned behaviors require practice. And if you backslide, even as I did today, remind yourself, forgive yourself, and practice some more.

I have been asked if I have advice to give. Yes, I have. Read every scrap of information about heart disease. So much is being published today, reported in the press, radio and TV that one can begin to understand warning signs, better ways of living, better ways of coping. You may have to wade through conflicting reports, but use your intelligence and a consultation with your doctor to sort it out. If I could have my wish, I would want women and men to be informed consumers of health care, investigate, question, question and question again, get two opinions—or three. Find a first class hospital. Don't be pushed around. Stick up for your rights. Be strong. Be courageous. And put on a teflon coat to protect yourself form taking it too much to heart.

And if you can, find out who you are and how you feel as early as possible in your life, learn to express your feelings and needs in relation to those in your circle. Try to learn to love yourself. Try to love yourself enough to take care of yourself. And love someone. Love life.

For all the danger I went through, I would not have missed the growth and spirituality I have enjoyed since my heart attack. God has been good to me. I know I have been a lucky woman with a continuing wonderful life.

I am still curious, still wanting to spread my arms to the landscape and to its creatures. And to life. To bring it all back together in a wholeness I could not have imagined.

Joe and I are sometimes tremulously close and in love. I find him growing more and more patient and philosophical, frequently more communicative than I. And forgiving of my increasingly exposed weaknesses.

I now stand guard at the gate to my heart and let no offending emotions enter.

afterword

As this book was being prepared for publication, the Journal of American Medical Association published the results of a Duke University five-year study concluding that mental stress is more dangerous to the heart than physical stress; that the way a person's body responds to mental stress can be a strong predictor of whether or not that person is vulnerable to cardiac events, even death.

Here was a gift, a gift to me. Here was clinical verification of what I had proved to myself about what had caused my heart attack. If this research had been published and widely circulated six years ago, I might never have undertaken my own research or written this book, never shared my story, and never committed myself to spreading the word.

Here was a gift to all women who had been shunted aside by physicians who said their heart disease symptoms were in their heads. The pains are real. They are in your heart.

Patients who displayed mental stress-induced ischemia had almost three times the risk ratio of having a cardiac event or of dying compared with patients who did not exhibit mental stress-induced ischemia, (blockage of the coronary arteries, resulting in insufficient blood and oxygen reaching the heart muscle.)

The authors write that this mental stress-induced heart pain predicts a heart event more strongly than an exercise-induced test and suggest that mental stress testing might complement traditional exercise stress testing in selected individuals.

Most of us know a little about exercise stress testing either on a treadmill or a bicycle; some of us have learned about a laboratory exercise stress test where nuclear tracers are injected and the patient's heart function is scanned and photographed.

In this study, five three-minute mental stress tests were administered: (1) mental arithmetic—patients were asked to perform a series of serial additions with encouragement and to perform calculations as quickly as possible; (2) public speaking—patients were asked to give a speech on a current-event topic to an audience of observers after one minute of preparation, and subjects were told that their speech would be evaluated; (3) mirror trace—subjects were asked to outline a star from its reflection in a mirror as quickly as possible; (4) reading aloud, with the stress of being evaluated, as in the speech-task, speakers read easy-to-read and neutral passages, from Readers Digest or North Carolina Wildlife; and (5) type "A" structured interview, which lasted up to twenty minutes with a six-minute rest period between each test.

After a twenty-minute rest period, all patients underwent exercise testing on a bicycle ergometer.

On the basis of their studies, the researchers recommend that it might be particularly appropriate to conduct future research to determine the effectiveness of stress management intervention for patients who exhibit stress-induced heart pain.

So, there it is. I am happy to have endured the pain of discovery through my own personal soul-searching. When I began, this study and others like it were just underway. But this study demonstrates how stress can be induced in a clinical setting and what damage it can do to your heart. I discovered this myself without benefit of a clinical test.

I am happy to share this with women—as well as men. it only increases my wish to shout again: TAKE CARE OF YOURSELVES. PAY ATTENTION. LIVE.

And live I do. Joe and I have just renewed our marriage vows at our fiftieth wedding anniversary.

Mickey Wapner

selected bibliography

BOOKS AND PAMPHLETS

Cedars-Sinai Medical Center-Department of Thoracic and Cardiovascular Surgery, *Heart to Heart.* (Postoperative Manual)
Cousins, Norman, *Anatomy of an Illness as Perceived by the Patient.* New York: W.W. Norton & company, 1979.
Douglas, Pamela S., M.D., *Heart Disease in Women.* Philadelphia: F.A. Davis Company, 1989.
Dorff, Elliot N., *Knowing God: Jewish Journeys to the Unknowable.* New Jersey: Jason Aronson Inc., 1992
Eliot, Robert S., M.D., And Dennis L. Breo, *Is it Worth Dying For? A Self-Assessment Program to Make Stress Work for You, Not Against You.* New York: A Bantam Book, 1989.
Ginsburg, Helen L., *From the Heart—Overcoming the Physical and Mental Trauma of Open Heart Surgery.* An Unpublished Manuscript, 1987
Goldberger, Leo, and Shlomo Breznitz, *Handbook of Stress—Theoretical and Clinical Aspects.* New York: The Free Press, 1993.
Karpman, Harold L., M.D., F.A.C.C., F.A.C.P., *Preventing Silent Heart Disease.* New York: Crown Publishers, Inc., 1989.
Klieman, Charles, M.D., and Kevin Orsborn, *If It Runs in Your Family—Heart Disease Reducing Your Risk.* Bantam Books, 1991.
Legato, Marianne J., M.D., and Coleman, Carol, *The Female Heart.* New York: Simon & Schuster, 1991.
McGoon, Michael D., M.D., *Mayo Clinic—Heart Book.* New York: William Morrow & Company, Inc., 1993.
Meier, Rabbi Levi, Ph.D., *Jewish Values in Health and Medicine.* Maryland: University Press of America, Inc., 1991
Ornish, Dean, M.D., *Dr. Dean Ornish's Program for Reversing Heart Disease.* New York: Random House, 1990.

Pashkow, Frederick J., M.D. and Charlotte Libov, *The Woman's Heart Book—The Complete Guide to Keeping Your Heart Healthy and What to Do If Things Go Wrong.* New York: Dutton, 1993.
Sandmaier, Marian, *The Healthy Heart Handbook.* National Heart, Lung, and Blood Institute: NIH Publication No. 92-2720, 1992
Selye, Hans, M.D., *The Stress of Life.* New York: McGraw-Hill Book Co., 1984
Sheehy, Gail, *The Silent Passage.* New York: Random House, 1991.
Williams, Redford, M.D., and Virginia Williams, Ph.D., *Anger Kills—Seventeen Strategies for Controlling the Hostility That Can Harm Your Health.* New York: Times Book, Random House, 1993.

JOURNAL ARTICLES/CONFERENCES/RESEARCH PAPERS

Ayanian, John Z., M.D., M.P.P., and Arnold M. Epstein, M.D., M.A., "Differences in the Use of Procedures Between Women and Men Hospitalized for Coronary Heart Disease," *New England Journal of Medicine,* Vol. 325, No. 4 (July 25, 1991), 221–30
"Conference on Women, Behavior and Cardiovascular Disease," *National Heart, Lung, and Blood Institute,* (September 25–27, 1991), Chevy Chase, Maryland.
Gordon, Dan, "Women's Health—Finally in the Research Picture," *UCLA Public Health,* Vol. 12, No. 1 (Spring/Summer 1993).
"Heart Disease: Women at Risk," *Consumer Reports,* Vol. 58, No. 5 (May 1993), 300–304.
Journal of the American Medical Association (JAMA), June 5, 1996. "Mental Stress-Induced Myocardial Ischemia and Cardiac Events."
Lehrman, Nathaniel S., M.D., "Pleasure Heals—the Role of Social Pleasure—Love in It's Broadest Sense—in Medical Practice," *Commentary, Arch Intern Med,* Vol. 153 (April 26, 1993), 929–934.
National Institutes of Health *Opportunities for Research on Women's Health,* (September 4–6, 1991), Hunt Valley, Maryland.

Interviews with:

Bairey-Merz, C. Noel, M.D.
  Medical Director of Preventive and Rehabilitative Cardiac Center of Cedars-Sinai Medical Center, Los Angeles
Blanche, Carlos, M.D.
  Associate Surgeon of the Dept. Of Cardiothoracic Surgery and Co-Director of Heart Transplant Program Cedar-Sinai Medical Center, Los Angeles
Bussell, John, M.D.
  Anesthesiologist, Cedars-Sinai Medical Center, Los Angeles
Friedman, Arnold, M.D.
  Anesthesiologist, Cedars-Sinai Medical Center, Los Angeles
Gray, Richard, M.D.
  Cardiologist
  Dean of Medical School, University of North Dakota
Hickey, Ann, M.D.
  Cardiologist, Cedars-Sinai Medical Center, Los Angeles
Jameson, Grace, M.D.
  Psychiatrist
  Professor, University of Texas Medical School, Galveston
Kahn-Rose, Robert, M.D.
  Psychiatrist, Memory Specialist
Lebe, Doryann, M.D.
  Psychiatrist
Mandel, William, M.D.
  Cardiologist
Marcus, Harold, M.D.
  Cardiologist
Matloff, Jack, M.D.
  Chairman of Cardiothoracic Surgery, Cedars-Sinai Medical Center, Los Angeles
Stokol, Colin, M.D.
  Neurologist
Uman, Stephen, M.D.
  Infectious Disease